Praise for *A Plant-Ric*

"When we really connect with the shocking reality, the cruelty and the disregard for beautiful sentient creatures when we choose to eat them, we are colluding not only with their destruction but also the destruction of our planet and ourselves. This book describes in a beautiful way why it doesn't have to be this way, that by deciding to be an ethical vegan you are choosing kindness and compassion over cruelty and indifference. What's not to like? Read this book and you'll see what I mean." - **Peter Egan, actor and animal advocate**

"Dr Rebecca Jones writes with the clarity of a clinician, the heart of a mother, and the conviction of a campaigner. I came to this book as a non-vegan, but also as someone who cares deeply about health, equity, and the future of our planet. Rebecca's writing is accessible, evidence-led, and refreshingly non-judgmental. What I took from A Plant-Rich Life is that this isn't just a book about food... it's a compassionate, courageous call to live more kindly. Whatever your starting point, it will meet you there." - **Dr Nikita Kanani MBE**

"A beautifully written, practical, and inspiring guide to living with compassion for all beings. Rebecca shows us that a plant-rich life is not only good for our health and the planet, but also deeply fulfilling." - **Dr Shireen Kassam, Founder and Director of Plant-Based Health Professionals UK**

"This is a much needed book explaining why veganism is such an important value system, and crucially explaining in simple yet informed terms how veganism can be embraced with vitality. The book provides both reassurance and hope for the future; it should be read by omnivores and vegans alike to help create a kinder world." - **Dr Gemma Newman, GP and author of 'The Plant Power Doctor' and 'Get Well, Stay Well.'**

"In A Plant-Rich Life, Dr Rebecca Jones blends science, compassion, and practical advice into an inspiring guide for anyone wanting to thrive. Her evidence-based approach shows how a plant-rich diet can nourish your body, boost overall well-being, and benefit the planet - all at the same time". - **Dr Alan Desmond, NHS gastroenterologist and author**

"Clear, compassionate, and courageously evidence-led, A Plant-Rich Life is the roadmap so many of us have been waiting for. Rebecca meets readers where they are, with science, sanity, and warmth, and turns plant-based living into something practical, joyful, and sustainable. It's a friendly, non-judgmental, evidence-based companion for anyone ready to embrace a kinder, healthier way of living." - **Robbie Lockie, Founder foodfacts.org & Plant Based News**

"This book has given me a much needed wake-up call. As a non-vegan, it's made me look at important things in a kinder and more honest way - my health, animal welfare and the survival of the planet." - **Dr Caroline Walker, The Joyful Doctor**

"Dr Rebecca Jones makes a fantastic case for veganism. Not only does she explore the main reasons to adopt this way of living, but she also provides practical insights into approaching making the change. She combines hard evidence with her own personal experiences through the lens of an NHS doctor, a mother, and a human who cares deeply for the state of the world. A must read for anyone curious about veganism or even for those already adopting a plant-based diet who want to strengthen their own knowledge." - **Dr Minil Patel, NHS GP and Lifestyle Medic**

A Plant-Rich Life

To Saffron
Happy Readers!
Best wishes,
Dr Rebecca :)

Print ISBN 978-1-0681630-0-5

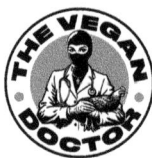

A Plant-Rich Life

Dr Rebecca E. Jones

For my love, S, who has always made me feel braver.

CONTENTS

Introduction

The idea of *The Vegan Doctor* was born in early 2017, just a few months after I transitioned to veganism. I had dabbled with plant-based eating in the past, but it was Veganuary 2017 that really cemented my decision to live a fully vegan lifestyle. What I soon came to appreciate is that it's really frustrating to be vegan in a non-vegan world. To some degree, I did expect this. What I didn't expect, however, was just how frustrating it was going to be to work as a vegan doctor in a non-vegan world, and in a *very* non-vegan profession.

My veganism didn't come completely out of the blue; I was brought up in various stages towards vegetarianism, and my parents were completely against most red meat since I was a toddler. In fact, I don't remember eating beef or lamb at all. I'd love to share the story of how they came to this decision to stop eating it, as it really is quite lovely.

My dad's side of the family are from Devon, and we would travel there most years for a holiday with relatives. My mum had recently had surgery to her foot just prior to one of these trips. This wasn't unusual for her, because she'd had a traumatic injury before I was born, so it wasn't so out of the ordinary for my mum to be wearing a plaster cast on her foot. One afternoon, we went for a stroll down a country lane, my mum walking slowly on her immobilised foot, pushing my baby sister in a buggy, and my dad walking with me, or perhaps carrying me on his shoulders. Mum's foot began to ache and so we stopped for a rest at a farm gate. Here, she sought some relief by raising her leg and placing her foot on the gate. At that moment, a herd of curious cows wandered over to see what was going on. As many people would, my mum feared what would happen next. But, encouraged by my dad, who told her that the cow wouldn't hurt her, she apprehensively left her foot where it was, and one gorgeous creature began licking the toes that were sticking out of her plaster cast! That tender interaction between my mum and the cow started our family on a whole new trajectory. One that has helped form the person I am today.

That evening was to be my mum's turn to cook for all the family. My parents had previously been shopping for the ingredients for a spaghetti bolognese, and although my mum did manage to cook for everyone else, after their encounter neither her nor my dad could stomach even the idea of eating beef mince. So it was spaghetti pomodoro for our dinner, and a future of vegetarianism and veganism for the four of us.

A few years later pork went, too. Unlike many vegans, I never particularly missed bacon, though, and I've never understood the whole 'Mmm, bacon' thing. The seed for giving up all red meat was really sown when my dad took me and my sister to the cinema to watch *Babe*, and he ended up falling in love with pigs. Interestingly, did you know that James Cromwell, the actor who played the farmer in the movie, turned vegan and became an animal rights activist because of his experience working with the animals on set? Not long after our trip to the cinema, my dad watched a documentary about the lives of pigs, and after witnessing just how intelligent they are, he decided that he could no longer eat pork, and the rest of the family followed. It took a bit longer for fish and chicken to go, but I got there, eventually.

I was lucky to be guided by compassionate parents who passed their ideas on to me. As a family we gradually became a bit more vegetarian every year, but were often at different stages of the transition. I remember as a teenager that my mum became a vegan, and I really did give it a try shortly after her. Unfortunately, I struggled and it didn't last. Over the next few years there were other attempts, sometimes half-hearted ones; for example, the time when I foolishly convinced myself that goat's cheese was kinder than cow's milk cheese. But I always seemed to fall back to being vegetarian. There were even months at a time when I went back to fish and sometimes chicken, but the guilt of eating sentient beings soon reared its head, and I would stop and return to vegetarianism.

After years of mumbling 'Sorry, Mum', as I tucked into a slice of cheese-on-toast or something similar in front of her and made proclamations of being a 'cheese hound', it suddenly dawned on me that the vegan message she had been gently trying to give to me was the *truth*. I had my lightbulb moment, and I haven't looked back. No one particular thing happened to trigger this. There was no epiphany. I was just sat on my sofa eating pasta topped with grated cheese when I suddenly felt like I really shouldn't be eating it.

Life as a vegan now is very different to when my mum's generation of vegans first signed up. We take for granted all of the meat-replacement products and dairy alternatives that often help us transition to veganism. But these substitutes aren't the only difference. The world is a much smaller place, and our access to world foods and interesting grains, pulses and spices has never been easier. I often think about how difficult it must have been for those vegans who went before us, thirty or even fifty years ago. They deserve so much of our thanks and respect.

In the end I found the change rather easy, but I guess that's because I was already vegetarian, and meat had never been a staple in my diet. However, when I joined various Facebook pages and forums, I soon realised that others were struggling with the transition.

There were plenty of other vegans who could help them with useful suggestions of meat replacements and shopping list ideas, but one area that was seriously lacking in good advice was the world of medicine. There were complaints of ignorant healthcare professionals advising vegans that their lifestyles were dangerous and unsustainable, and there were many doctors who just didn't understand what it meant.

That's when I had the idea for *The Vegan Doctor*. I understood that I was in a unique position, being a GP *and* an ethical vegan. So I started blogging, and I took myself back to university to study for a postgraduate diploma in Clinical Nutrition, equipping myself with as much knowledge as possible. The topics I started writing about varied from nutritional advice and myth-busting articles, to helping vegans to know when to see their GP.

Thankfully, things have changed in the last couple of years. There are some really great plant-based physicians who have written books, or have popular social media accounts. This book is slightly different, however; my focus isn't solely on the use of a plant-based diet for health, but rather how to retain and optimise health whilst making the ethical and moral choice to be vegan. But I also acknowledge that those choices we make are an important part of our wellbeing, because our health and the natural world are very interconnected. Together, we will explore all of these reasons; some well-known, and others that might be new to you.

The most significant change that I noticed after transitioning was a huge increase in my interest in food and cooking. I think many vegans feel like this, and cooking becomes exciting. Whether it's veganising familiar dishes, or learning about pulses, grains and veggies that you might not have cooked with before, I think we're all on a quest for variety. I'd never spent so much time making new dishes, and photographing my food! I'm so passionate about all aspects of veganism that I wanted to put everything that I have learned into one place to help you feel confident making the changes necessary to achieve your vegan life.

I'm going to tell you all of the compelling reasons why you should consider living a plant-rich life. I'm going to reassure you that it's safe to make the transition, with lots of nutrition guidance, and then I'll show you how to get started. My recipes will help you to feed yourself and your family delicious vegan food that's full of goodness, and tasty enough to keep you on track with your new vegan journey. You might even convince a few sceptics with these dishes!

Please think of this book, and me, if you like, as a good friend helping to make this big, important change; a source that you can trust to give you balanced, non-judgmental, evidence-based information. And you can come back to us time and time again, whenever you need to remind yourself of why you've made these choices, or you are having a bit of a wobble.

I wish you all the luck in the world with your new plant-rich life. But I'm also really, really excited for you. You've got a beautiful new way of living ahead of you. One that is tastier, healthier, and kinder. And you are going to feel so much better for it.

Thank you for reading,

Rebecca, The Vegan Doctor

WHY VEGANISM?

1

Vegan for the Animals

'There is no fundamental difference between man and animals in their ability to feel pleasure and pain, happiness, and misery.' — Charles Darwin

Thinking about animal rights can be painful, and uncomfortable. Even if we don't realise it, we often avoid dialogues around this, or avoid looking at anything depicting what happens to animals. But many people only think about animal cruelty as applying to cats, dogs, and other domestic pets. Vegans take that one step further and apply the same principles to farmed animals that omnivores eat. In fact, I believe that the reason most people don't really like vegans, or make jokes about how we can't help talking about veganism, is because we reveal an uncomfortable truth. We show you and tell you about the things you don't really want to see and hear. Because the things that happen to these animals really is horrific, and once you've seen these things, you can't unlearn them. It's no coincidence that slaughterhouses are located where nobody goes.

'For the animals', often abbreviated on social media to FTA, was the reason I first became vegan, and while my research and learning has led me to the position of believing that veganism is also essential to safeguard the future health of humanity as a whole, and to protect the earth and all of its inhabitants, vegan FTA will always be the most important to me. I am so happy that you have taken the really difficult and brave step to explore veganism, and to read about what most people don't even want to consider: the rights of animals to live and be free. However, if this feels like too much right now, or you don't think the words in this chapter will appeal to you as an important reason to start living plant-based, then please head to the next chapter, and come back when you feel ready. Maybe learning about what the meat and dairy industry are doing to our earth, or how plants are better for your health might help you to make the transition a little more easily. But please do come back. Once we know all of the reasons, and start connecting them, becoming vegan is a very easy decision to make. And as you'll soon read, it is all about those connections.

The fact that I am a traditionally trained clinical doctor using the word vegan over plant-based should tell you all you need to know about my motivations. While the term plant-based pretty much perfectly describes how I and most other vegans eat, that's about all it does describe. As you will be starting to realise, veganism is about so much more than what we put into our mouths. I think about my veganism not just when I'm shopping, cooking and eating, but also when I'm buying our household cleaning products, clothing my children, and planning our holidays and days out. It's a way of life, not a diet. And animal rights is where it all started for me, so out of all the reasons for choosing this plant-rich life, this chapter is the one that is closest to my heart.

The Vegan Society defines veganism as:

'a philosophy and way of living which seeks to exclude – as far as is possible and practicable – all forms of exploitation of, and cruelty to, animals for food, clothing or any other purpose; and by extension, pro-

motes the development and use of animal-free alternatives for the benefit of animals, humans and the environment. In dietary terms it denotes the practice of dispensing with all products derived wholly or partly from animals.'

I've always been a bit stubborn about calling myself The Vegan Doctor, not The Plant-Based Doctor, for all of the reasons I have already given. And this has often been questioned by colleagues and supporters who have suggested that I might be more acceptable or palatable to readers if I were to change my name. I've also been heavily criticised by other vegans for not 'staying in my lane' online, sharing information about how veganism affects more than just the rights and lives of non-human animals. But I was recently looking at the definition from the Vegan Society again when I was preparing a presentation about living a plant-rich life. And despite having read it so many times, I suddenly saw something that hadn't registered with me before: 'for the benefit of animals, humans and the environment'. Even the definition from the Vegan Society itself states that veganism is for the benefit of all – for humans and the environment, as well as the animals. Despite many staunch vegans arguing that I shouldn't be discussing health benefits and environmental impacts under the name of The Vegan Doctor, all three reasons are encompassed by the original definition. So I guess you could argue that pushing the vegan agenda for health and the planet does fit with my identity as a vegan doctor over a merely plant-based one! But, why? What would the problem be? Why is veganism in its simplest definition so important to me?

Let's firstly clarify a few things: vegans don't consume any animal-derived foods, wouldn't allow any animal ingredients in their household or self-care products, wouldn't wear any leather, wool or silk, and would avoid any products that had been tested on, or had utilised animals anywhere in their production. It sounds a lot, doesn't it? But once you get into a routine with it, it really does become quite normal. And there are so many more truly vegan and cruelty-free products on the market now, that it really isn't too difficult. I'll tell you more about that later in the book.

Plant-based, on the other hand, defines a diet. Whilst all vegans are plant-based, not all plant-based people are vegan. Some people are more strictly plant-based, and will not eat any animal products at all, but they may not consider what's in their lotions and potions at home, and might not avoid things that have been animal tested. Some people who call themselves plant-based are more like 'plant-dominant' with their diet, meaning they're mostly plant-based, but might eat honey, or have occasional portions of meat, fish, eggs or dairy.

At the end of the day, the differences between how we define ourselves shouldn't really matter. Some people might call themselves plant-based and be doing it for the environment, others might call themselves vegan but be doing it only for their health. In my view, as long as fewer animals are being harmed, this is a positive thing. Of course I want **no** animals at all to be exploited by humans, so every step towards a world that looks like this is wonderful. But I also want us all to be able to talk about veganism without the majority treating it like a dirty word. Because it isn't, and those of us who believe that animals deserve equal rights to humans should be able to speak up and admit this, without fear of being laughed at, discriminated against, or treated as an outsider or a weirdo. So this is why I have always insisted on being known as a vegan doctor, not a plant-based one. I want the world to see that educated professionals, who have assessed the evidence, and live and work as a valuable member of society can be vegan, with no shame, helping to promote the vegan cause.

I'm sure if you're reading this book, you will already know a bit about veganism as you will have had some curiosity or motivation to be thinking about it. But perhaps you are one of those people who is doing it for the planetary benefits, or maybe dabbling in plant-based eating for your health? So I'll tell you a little bit more about animal agriculture. Then, perhaps, the idea of 'vegan for the animals' might appeal to you too.

The Meat Industry

In the UK alone, 1.2 billion land animals are killed every year for food.[1] Can you even imagine a number that big? And each one of those animals was a sentient being, who was most likely factory farmed in wretched conditions before their untimely and terrifying death in a slaughterhouse. And I say untimely, because most of the animals that are slaughtered for food are just babies. Apart from the miserable life they live in the captivity of industrial farms, they also just don't want to die. What animal does? I have often heard it argued that we might be anthropomorphising animals when this is said. But even if we take all sentimentality out of our view of animals, we have to understand that they are sentient beings with a genetic drive to survive. So of course they'll fear the slaughterhouse killing floor, or the sounds of other animals being slaughtered, or the smell of spilled blood.

I don't even think it's that sentimental to go one step further and think about the fact that we *know* animals are sentient. Those with pets are well aware of the fact that animals have the capacity to be happy: in the UK we spend around £8bn per year on our furry friends.[2] We know that they are able to think and feel, and experience things happening around them. The only real difference is that they aren't able to use verbal language to tell us how they are feeling. So perhaps we need to do better at reading their non-verbal language instead. Maybe then we'll be able to understand and accept how much pain and suffering we are putting them through in their short lives.

There's so much disconnect in how we live our lives; it applies in our relationships with one another, in a capitalist society that encourages us to value individualism, and between entire cultures and ethnicities who don't realise they have more in common with each other than not. We've even disconnected our bodies from our minds, failing to understand just how much they impact one another. But in this case the disconnect is from how and what we eat. Importantly, it's from *who* we eat. We'll discuss capitalism more later on in this book, but here it's relevant because it is the process of capitalism that has turned these animals, whose lives and bodies they have commodified, into mere products. People simply don't have to think about the origins of most of their foods, but I think this primarily applies to meat, either because it's been turned into something that doesn't really represent real food, like a sausage or a nugget, or because language like 'shoulder of lamb' has been so normalised in the context of food, that people don't consider that it really is a lamb's shoulder.

Or perhaps a person might be aware, but they don't care or have enough empathy for the animals a step down from us in the 'food chain'. They might think that a) it's natural, b) animals are lesser beings that don't require our compassion, or c) meat is necessary. As you'll discover in the 'Vegan for Health' chapter, meat is absolutely unnecessary for good health. In fact it contributes to poor health. And we're going to learn just how harmful it is to the environment. So let us just discuss the arguments why it isn't natural and why animals really do deserve our compassion.

Farming

Factory farming is a relatively new concept, introduced as an answer to ever growing demands of an ever growing human population. It's only since around the 1930s that animals have been farmed in such intensive conditions, when the slaughter of pigs became mechanised in the US.[3] This method of farming has crept into British agricultural practices, and a 2017 report from The Bureau of Investigative Journalism described that there were around 1700 intensive pig and chicken farms in the UK at that time.[4] That number has since grown, as has the number of animals kept crammed into small spaces. At the time of writing, there have been reports of avian flu spreading through farms in the US, and one farm had to cull all of their birds. Take a guess how many birds were on that one farm. OK, I'll tell you: 1.4 million. Yes, million. On one farm, all slaughtered in one go.

In some ways this is no surprise at all. The earth's human population is expected to reach 10 billion by 2050, and all of those people need to eat. If the majority are continuing to eat animals, of course those creatures are going to be kept in ever more cramped conditions, because there's just not enough space for all of those animals, and they will be slaughtered in ever increasing numbers to meet demand. But you can imagine what those conditions might look like, right? Cramped. Smelly. Infection-laden. Dark. So these animals who are so cruelly slaughtered, years before their expected natural lifespan, live hard and painful lives before they even get to that miserable end.

So normal has animal cruelty become, we can't even rely on regulatory bodies to keep farming conditions comfortable for the animals trapped within them. This was, questionably, always down to the RSPCA (Royal Society for the Prevention of Cruelty to Animals), but a recent article by the environmentalist and writer,

George Monbiot,[5] described the dreadful findings of a report by the charity Animal Rising.[6] They went to several 'RSPCA Assured' farms and found animals in the most appalling conditions. Quite apart from the fact that it is bizarre that an organisation dedicated to protecting animals and ensuring their welfare would be responsible for approving the conditions under which they are farmed and slaughtered, it is shameful that they haven't even succeeded at this. They have approved farms where what was happening to animals was so distressing that footage of their *living* conditions (not even the slaughter) was 'unwatchable'.

Whenever we talk about this, there is always somebody who argues that they eat grass-fed, organic beef, and other animals bred outdoors. Even if we could be safe in the knowledge that these animals really are bred more kindly, which we aren't, there are a number of significant flaws in these arguments. Firstly, no matter how those animals are farmed, they still end up being transported and slaughtered well before their time, and we'll read more below about why we can no longer justify these practices. But this method of farming is also unsustainable; apart from the fact that most people around the world won't be able to afford these expensive meats, resulting in a two-tier food system with only the rich eating meat, there are also considerable environmental concerns associated with grazing beef cows. We'll cover more about this in the 'Vegan for the Planet' chapter, but let's just say that grass-fed beef is not the answer.

Live transport

In the same way that most people who eat meat don't think about where (or who) their food came from, most people certainly don't think about how it got there. We know that thinking about slaughter is really unpleasant, and probably not conducive to an enjoyable meal. And we'll discuss this in more detail in the slaughter section below. But one stage of meat production that is often forgotten is that of the transportation of animals.

Animals need to be moved from one place to another. With farming being done on an industrial level, as we've already discussed, slaughter doesn't usually happen on the farm any more, like it might have done when farms were small and farmers knew each and every animal. Instead, animals are transported to an equally industrial abattoir. These animals aren't used to travelling. They are meant to be living out their lives in fields and forests. They're not meant to know what being in the back of a truck feels like.

Much like the conditions in factory farms, animals are crammed into the confined spaces of trucks and lorries, many of which don't have any air conditioning or water. Very worryingly, it's currently legal to allow animals to be moved in such vehicles for up to 8 hours without a break. As a human being, with access to my own flask of water, and whatever form of entertainment I choose, even I would struggle with 8 hours of travelling without a break. Where water is available, pigs can be transported for 24 hours continuously, with cows being given a break after 14 hours.[7] And the temperatures in these vehicles can be stifling when the weather is warm. How is it illegal to leave a dog in a hot car, prompting passers-by to smash windows and rescue them, but nobody is concerned about the fact that animals are transported to their death in extreme heat? In fact, every year millions of animals die from dehydration, extreme stress, starvation, injury and illness during transportation.[8] And what kind of world do we live in, when somebody who has the compassion to feed water to dehydrated animals on the back of a truck is arrested for doing so?[9]

Of course we should be considering the temperatures and access to water on these journeys, but what about the fact that it's just really stressful for animals to be moved from the place where they are bred onto a vehicle, which is a completely strange experience for them, and onward to the rest of the journey when they have never experienced travel before. If you have ever taken your dog or cat on a car journey, when they haven't spent much time in a car before, you have probably seen just how stressful this can get for them. What about when transport lorries crash or overturn? I'm regularly being shown online news stories about large numbers of cows and other victims who have had to be euthanised after being horribly injured when the truck carrying them collided with another vehicle or had overturned. It's also not infrequent that you see supposedly 'feel-good' stories about escapees from such trucks, who leap from the top of the back of a lorry to get away from the awful conditions inside, and their awaited fate. Imagine how dreadful things must be inside that van for an individual to feel safer jumping from a moving height to the unknown.

Slaughter

After the harrowing ride to the slaughterhouse, before they've even reached the awful ultimate event, the treatment of animals in the abattoir can often be really unpleasant, and sometimes downright sadistic.

Many people have convinced themselves that animals are killed 'humanely'. After all, how could you consume the flesh of someone that has been killed for your palate if you knew that it had suffered terribly? But I could argue that there is no such thing as humane slaughter. These animals don't want to die. They haven't sacrificed themselves for our eating pleasure. Instead, they experience fear and anxiety, as they approach the site of their slaughter, often hearing the cries of the animals meeting their end up ahead, smelling the scents of blood, faeces and death. Sir Paul McCartney has famously said that 'If slaughterhouses had glass walls, everybody would be vegetarian.' I suspect he's right. We are so disconnected from the products that we're eating, that we don't consider the origin of the piece of meat sitting on our plate. We don't think about the pain and suffering that animal might have gone through before they were butchered and made to look more like food. If we did, we might, in-deed, lose our appetites.

So what does happen in the slaughterhouse? We're rarely shown, and most of us would rather not see. But as we're talking about all the reasons to be vegan, let's be candid. I apologise for the descriptions I'm about to make of slaughter, but if we are to consider going vegan because we believe that animals deserve better, then we must bear witness to what they suffer. It's only by being open-minded, and seeing how things are really done, that we can begin to change them, and make them better. So please stay with me, while we read about what these animals endure.

Cows and sheep

Large animals like cows, sheep and pigs, are required to be stunned, and for cows and sheep this means they are usually shot with a bolt in or through the head to knock them out. They are then strung up to a pulley system where they move along a conveyer belt style system to have their throats cut. They are bled, which is the actual mode of slaughter. Unfortunately, it isn't completely unheard of for an animal to have not been stunned properly, or for them to regain consciousness before or during the slaughter process, meaning they might experience much or all of this. After death, they move on to the next slaughterhouse worker who will skin, disembowel and dis-member them. Sadly, I have heard stories of animals not yet being dead before this process is started too, and isn't unheard of that an unborn calf spills out from a cow's body when she is being disembowelled.

For me, this is the stuff of horror movies. But honestly, I think it's probably the same for most of us, vegan or not. If we were to stop and think about this happening to a sentient being during the process of meat production, perhaps more of us would stop eating them. But cognitive dissonance allows many of us to keep on consuming meat despite knowing deep down that the way that food reached our plates isn't just wrong, it's completely unethical.

Pigs

The method of stunning for pigs is a bit different: they are either gassed with carbon dioxide (CO_2) or they are soaked and electrocuted. The end result should be the same, that they should be rendered unconscious, but up to a third of pigs are still fully conscious when they are killed.[10] The method of slaughter is the same as with cows: they are strung up and have their throats cut, then are allowed to bleed out until they die. After this they are dipped into boiling water to scald off their hair. They then go through a similar process of dismemberment and disembowelment.

The same problems that we read about with cows and sheep during the slaughter process can occur with pigs. Stunning might not occur properly, meaning that they might also be conscious when they are dipped into the scalding water. How humane is the method of gassing is also questionable. Whilst stunning is meant to be a way of making slaughter kinder, or more humane, being gassed with

CO_2 is a painful, frightening experience, which has been deemed to be 'incompatible with pig welfare'.[11]

Chickens and other birds

Chickens are also stunned by either being gassed or electrocuted. When gassed they are put into crates, and transferred to a chamber filled with toxic gas, but this can also be used as the mode of slaughter, by leaving them in there until they die. For electrocution, they are shackled upside down by their legs to a conveyer system that moves them to an electrified bath. They are completely conscious until the moment their heads hit the water, when they become stunned, before being moved further along to a mechanical method of throat cutting, which is the cause of death. The shackling itself is rough and painful, and can cause fractures of the bones in their legs. Another problem is that the birds are able to dodge the electrified water, meaning that they can be conscious during slaughter, which itself can also be unsuccessful, meaning they can, like pigs, end up in a bath of scalding water alive.

And what about the ages at which these creatures are slaughtered? They are usually killed when they are barely out of infancy. Where their natural life span would be up to around 20 years, beef cows are killed at 11 or 12 months. And chickens, who would ordinarily live until around 5–10 years old are usually just about 6 weeks old when they make it onto the dinner plate. That's no age at all, is it? Most people don't even think about the fact that lamb is called lamb, the name for a *baby* sheep, because that's what it is: a baby. They are usually slaughtered at 3 to 6 months old, just a fraction of their 12-year life expectancy. Pigs, who would usually live until about 15 years old, are slaughtered at around 6 months old.

Fishing

It's not just land animals that are horribly exploited. Many people just don't think of fish as 'meat'. There is even a sub-type of vegetarian called 'pesco-vegetarian'. Even in the most basic terms, I find this bizarre. We know fish are sentient, but is it really just the case that because we can't see them every day, that we completely disregard the lives of fish as having any meaning at all?

The fishing industry kills trillions of fish globally, every year. Literally trillions. I can't even comprehend that number. Never mind the devastating effect that pulling that many creatures from the oceans has on our environment, which we will discuss in more detail later, but, as if it even needed to be questioned, fish have also been shown to be sentient.[12] They live rich lives, and have relationships, and perhaps most importantly, they feel pain. Once again though, it's not just the killing of these creatures that is so unjust. It is also the conditions in industrial farms, which we have already discussed earlier for land animals. But, many people don't realise that fish are farmed, and that this is usually in very unnatural, cramped conditions, rife with disease and injury.

The Dairy Industry

But surely vegetarianism would fix any problems with all of the above, wouldn't it? If everybody was vegetarian, then couldn't we avoid the factory farming and the slaughter? Well no, not really. We haven't even got to the problems with the dairy and egg industries yet.

In my opinion, and I think that of most vegans, the dairy industry is far more inhumane than the meat industry, yet it often gets overlooked by compassionate vegetarians, and completely ignored by everybody else. Again, what you can't see can't hurt you, right? But the hidden realities of dairy farming are just awful. You can't make milk without pregnancy. That's a simple, biological fact, despite the fact that many milk drinkers and farmers will dispute it. So, the dairy industry relies on a continuous cycle of forced insemination, pregnancy, birth, and removal of the newborn. Over and over again. Cruelties inflicted on both a mother and her newborn, over and over.

Let's consider the dairy cow, or the mother, first. In the last few years I have become a mother, and I now know what that maternal instinct to protect your offspring feels like. I'm not arrogant or ignorant enough to think that it feels any different for me because I'm a human animal. I know that most of my instincts and behaviours are shared with other mammals. I just know how to intellectualise these things and reflect upon them. The idea of having my baby taken from me, and then being milked whilst going through the emotional agony of being in the postnatal state without my offspring, is just devastating. And, even worse than that? Being made to do it over and over again until I'm physically exhausted. But humans have lost our connection with so many things: with other animals, our place in nature, our own bodies and their functions. If we stopped and truly thought about what we're doing to a dairy cow, could we really justify the pain and suffering she goes through when oat milk tastes just as good and contains all the healthy nutrients without the harmful saturated fat and carcinogens?

So what is it that we put cows through? Obviously insemination occurs without any kind of consent. One might laugh at the idea of a cow giving consent. But why not? On some level, there will be some kind of consent given which allows a male cow access to her for the purpose of procreation – even if this is as simple as a passive implied consent that she allows penetration to go ahead. But a cow doesn't have any awareness of the concept of artificial insemination to allow it, or not. It also looks like it's quite an unpleasant experience. Just to make sure that I didn't give you any false information when I wrote a description of this, I searched 'what happens to a cow during insemination'. I found detailed instructions on a website called Farmers Weekly,[13] which explains that you begin by making sure the cow is restrained. That really tells you everything you need to know, doesn't it?

What I confirmed is that the process really is as horrible as I had believed; the cow's back passage will be penetrated with a farmer's hand and arm to locate her cervix, and he pushes down on her vagina with that elbow before inserting a device (they call it a gun), which contains semen, into the vagina with the other hand. I've already made the connection between human and cow mothers, but here's another one. A cow is pregnant for around 9 months, just like us. But when her gestational period is over, she won't have a joyful meeting with her baby. Well, she might but it's likely to be short-lived. The dairy industry tends to remove the calf within 24 hours. We'll find out a little later what happens to the calf in this situation.

Pregnancy for mammals means milk. Well, that's the whole reason for insemination, pregnancy and removing a calf, isn't it? But how do we get it? Dairy cows will spend a significant portion of each day hooked up to a milking machine. Anybody who has breast-fed and tried to use a breast pump will tell you this is unlikely to be a pleasant experience. But not only is it unnatural and intrusive, it's also uncomfortable. And lactation isn't always a straightforward process. Even the most experienced of breast(/chest)feeders will be susceptible to mastitis, a nasty infection in the milk-engorged breast, which can quickly lead to sepsis, and is renowned for being very painful. Up to a quarter of all dairy cows will experience at least one episode of mastitis in any given year,[14] meaning they'll be in pain, and will require antibiotics. But the machinery itself also causes harm. They can cause trauma, resulting in lacerations to the teats, and this happens quite routinely. I can only imagine, as a current breastfeeder, how painful this must be. As you can probably imagine by these descriptions of industrialised methods of milking, most dairy cows spend their lives indoors, in huge sheds, hundreds of cows to each. This is a stark contrast to the imagined lives of dairy cows by many people who just don't understand the reality. There is no grazing on luscious green fields, and on-site churning of milk by the farmer's wife.

After all of this exhausting work, cows don't get to rest. They repeat the cycle time and time again, until they are no longer producing enough milk to be profitable. At this point they are slaughtered. This will be the reality for the 1.85 million cows in the UK,[15] but all of this happens out of the view of the general public. So none of us really has to think about where our cheese comes from – that the cheese you enjoy, without a second thought, guilt free, only exists because of the removal of a calf from its mother who will be slaughtered for its meat at just a few weeks old, if it even survives that long. So let's talk about the calf's journey. The baby in this dyad. Or 'waste', as they are seen in the dairy industry.

I've lost count of the number of videos I've seen of distressed female cows chasing after a cart containing her newborn, or tackling a farmer that's trying to remove them. Or photos of rows and rows of sheds each containing a calf who is being kept in a confined space to keep its meat in the right condition for sale as veal, whilst calling for its mother. And anyone who lives near a dairy farm will tell you about the cries of both mother and baby after they are separated. But none of this is surprising. Nature has designed this bond between mother and baby to be strong. It's not imagined by us as humans, and we're no different. We're mammals. We feel the same as other mothers. The only 'comfort' is that a mother cow will never know what her baby will go through.

A calf, once removed from the mother who just birthed them, will be either shot immediately, or taken to a small shed and raised for veal until they are 5 or 6 months old. Then they will be slaughtered, enduring the awful conditions of the slaughterhouse already described. How dreadful is it that a baby can be exposed to this, and after 6 long months of isolation and longing for its mother. If they are not slaughtered for veal, then they might make it to a year when they are killed for beef; and if they survive beyond this, it's because they are female, and so put back into the dairy industry to endure their mother's fate.

I wonder if dairy was an essential part of the human diet, would I be able to accept any of what I've just described? I think once you know, it's hard to overlook the cruelty and inhumanity of what we do to cows. But the reality is that we absolutely do not need to drink milk, or use dairy products, and this makes it all the worse. Milk is a fluid produced for infants, and as for infant cows, they don't even get to drink their mother's milk. No other animal on this earth drinks milk beyond childhood. And neither should we.

Take lactose intolerance as a perfect example of why we shouldn't be drinking milk. I'll touch on lactose intolerance a bit more in the 'Vegan for Social Justice' chapter, but one important bit of information we can borrow from there, is that 65% of the world's population is unable to properly digest lactose, a sugar found in milk. It's rather logical, when you really think about it, that we should no longer need to be able to digest lactose. If milk is meant for babies, then why would we be able to? The enzyme which breaks lactose down is called lactase, and babies readily produce plenty of it. As an infant ages, the amount of lactase they make reduces, ready for the time when they will no longer rely on their mother's milk for nutrition.

But humans, as weird as we are, have somehow decided that we require milk beyond the usual age of weaning. Not our mother's milk though, no. That would be just too strange. Of course only the milk of another's mother will do. Cow, sheep or goat is just fine. Just as long as it's not human, the only kind of animal whose milk our bodies were evolved to consume.

We also have to wonder just why we're so obsessed with milk. I'll explain more in the 'Vegan for Health' chapter about the risks of dairy for human health, but what I can tell you is that there are many studies that have shown that dairy is *not* essential for healthy bones. Not only this, but fortified alternatives like oat and soya milk provide pretty much the same profile of micronutrients like calcium, vitamin D and iodine, whilst cutting out the harmful saturated fat. They also taste delicious, and don't lead to the same inflammatory effects as dairy milk, which can cause so much harm to human health. If you could prevent such abject cruelties like those inflicted in the dairy industry by drinking something that is, in fact, healthier, why would you even give it a second thought?

Eggs

Eggs can also seem rather harmless until you really delve into what's going on in that industry. Chickens are pretty much unrecognisable as a natural animal, and their behaviours have been heavily manipulated. Wild hens would usually produce around 20 eggs per year, but an industrial environment leads them to lay 300 per year, in conditions that are often extremely cramped, where their beaks may be painfully trimmed, and again where they are disposed of once no longer laying, cutting their lives short.

Many people are led to believe that free range eggs are kinder, or fairer; after all, wouldn't hens lay eggs anyway? Unfortunately, no matter whether you choose eggs from caged hens or free range, many of the cruelties enacted upon them happen no matter what their living situation is.

It's not just chickens that are bred for meat that have a shortened lifespan. Earlier in this chapter we learned that chickens in the wild live up to 10 years, but those trapped within the egg industry usually live for only 18 months. During their short life, instead of roaming, mooching around outdoors, and living in their natural hierarchy, caged hens are forced into cramped spaces where they are often pecked at, and live their lives in darkness and with high levels of stress.

The abject brutality to which chickens are exposed starts from the moment they hatch. Literally, from the moment they begin to exist, they are tipped onto a conveyor belt where they are moved to a person who will sex the chicks. Males are disposed of, seen only as waste. They will be either gassed or thrown into a macerator. It's unfathomable to imagine the experiences of these babies, who survive less than a day, to come to such a horrible end. But this happens to 40 million male chicks every year in the UK.[16] And the females who survive will never experience their mother. Much like with the dairy industry, we've completely removed the connection between these animals and their young. We've deprived them of the right to reproduce in a natural way – probably their only innate drive, beyond eating and surviving.

Again, much like the female cow, hens enter a harsh cycle of cruelty: forced egg production. They have the ends of their beaks trimmed to prevent them from hurting one another in their cramped living spaces, even if the chickens are destined for a free range-farm. This procedure is known to be painful and traumatic, and is done without any kind of anaesthesia or numbing. Egg-producing hens have been bred to be lightweight and frail, their health being sacrificed for efficient egg production. Their bones don't contain the usual quantity of minerals like calcium and phosphorus, instead being directed into the unnatural amount of eggs they produce. This leads to bone disease and pain.

We can't escape the fact that choosing free-range eggs won't prevent the deaths of millions of male chicks every year, nor the awful process of beak trimming that happens to every egg-producing hen. Free-range also doesn't necessarily mean that the hens live happy lives. Yes, they might have a little more space, but in reality this means that up to 9 hens can share one square metre, and this space is still often cramped, dark, and deprives the chickens of natural stimulation and social interactions. And while organic eggs might improve the welfare of hens trapped in the egg industry somewhat, this is often not as well regulated as you might be led to believe; living conditions can still be poor, and we can't escape the fact that male chicks are still slaughtered on their first day of life.

There is one way, of course, to prevent these things from happening, or at the very least to refuse to participate in them yourself: veganism. And when you can replace an egg in your baking with something as simple as a tablespoon of flax seeds or a spoonful of apple sauce, why would you choose the option of cruelty instead?

Vegan Take-Aways

Animals are here with us, not for us, and they deserve better than the short lives they are given in factory farms.

Humans don't need milk beyond infancy. Calves do need their mother's milk, and contact with her.

Animals killed for meat are done so in infancy; they are still babies.

Eating eggs means taking part in a system where male chicks are killed at birth, often by maceration.

1.2 billion animals are killed every year in the UK for food. Globally, it's 82 billion.

There is no such thing as humane slaughter. Animals have a natural drive towards survival, and feel fear and pain just as humans do.

2

Vegan for the Planet

'Livestock farming ranks . . . as one of the two most destructive industries on Earth. But because of those farmyard tales, reinforced by stories we're told as adults . . . we apply entirely different standards to it.' — George Monbiot

Soon after I became vegan for the animals, I learned more and more about the environmental impacts of animal agriculture. So it wasn't long before the environmental reasons for adopting a plant-based diet became almost as important as the animal welfare reasons for me. I've often thought that I would like my legacy to be that I leave the world just a little better than it was when I came into it. And now that I have children, I'm compelled to think about the state in which we will leave our home, the planet Earth, for the next generation. So I feel that I have *no other choice* than to follow a plant-based diet, not only because I care about animal welfare and rights, but also because I don't want to cause any more harm to this wonderful planet than my human presence on it already does.

We don't talk enough about the impact of animal agriculture on the planet, and the media certainly doesn't cover this sufficiently. We hear a lot about fossil fuels and travel, about carbon emissions and pollution. So let's talk about it now. What if I told you that agriculture is one of the leading causes of climate change, with practices related to animal agriculture, specifically, doing the most harm?[17] And it's not just greenhouse gas emissions. The animal agriculture industry affects the environment in so many different ways. Let's have a look at some of them.

Greenhouse Gas Emissions

When we talk about emissions, we're talking about greenhouse gases. These are atmospheric gases that raise the earth's temperature. This is why they're called 'greenhouse gases,' because they work to absorb waves of radiation from the sun, causing a rise in temperature. It's much like what happens in a greenhouse, causing it to create a warm atmosphere for growing tomatoes and other veggies.

These gases include carbon dioxide (CO_2), methane (CH_4) and nitrous oxide (N_2O). There are others, but these three are the gases whose increased volume in the earth's atmosphere have the most impact on global warming. Global warming is a concern because it will damage every ecosystem on earth, systems whose functions should be in a careful, beautiful balance. We are already looking at a situation where there is melting of the polar ice caps, rising sea levels and disastrous weather events, as well as mass extinction, human famines, and infectious disease outbreaks.

It sounds like a disaster movie, doesn't it? But it's real and it's already underway, all because of human behaviours. In fact, horrifyingly, scientists have argued that we are currently in the sixth mass extinction event, and that humans are responsible for it.[18]

Carbon dioxide

Carbon dioxide is the greenhouse gas which is most commonly produced by human activity by the burning of fossil fuels and through other industrial processes like deforestation and the agricultural degradation of soil. I'll cover land clearing and deforestation a little later, but they contribute to increased CO_2 emissions by removing trees and foliage that would usually store CO_2 which they have absorbed from the environment. If I can take you back to your primary school level biology for a moment, do you remember how plants and animals exchange oxygen and carbon dioxide?

When humans breathe, we take in oxygen from the environment, our bodies absorb it via the blood vessels around our lungs, and we expel the waste product of respiration, CO_2, back into the lungs from our circulatory system, and then breathe this out. This is called gaseous exchange. Plant life does something very similar, but almost in complete reverse, and as such, they use and store our waste CO_2, which would otherwise be floating freely in the atmosphere, contributing to the greenhouse effect. Which it does. Just stop and consider for one moment how incredible that symbiotic relationship is. Just how wonderful a job trees do for us, to keep our atmosphere just as we need it. It's amazing how connected our existence is to nature and the life all around us, but in forgetting this and not valuing the roles that other living beings on this planet have, we're losing that connection, and harming ourselves and everything on planet Earth. We have damaged this process so much that CO_2 levels are now 48% higher than when industrialisation began.[19]

Methane

Methane is produced by ruminants, which are animals that are herbivorous. This means that they extract the nutrients in their diet by fermentation. This process results in the production of methane in the form of belching and flatus (they're at it from both ends, basically!), which in the natural world, if it wasn't interfered with by humans, would likely balance itself out, as those animals would be part of a wider ecosystem. But as the ruminants include cows, sheep and goats, all of which humans farm and eat, you can imagine what an unnaturally high number of these animals might mean for atmospheric methane levels. Although they aren't ruminants, our industrial farming of pigs also contributes to the increase in atmospheric methane levels because the waste lagoons* on pig farms also produce this gas.

(*I always find it bizarre that something as disgusting as a pond or lake made solely from pig faeces could be given such a lovely sounding name as *lagoon*.)

Nitrous oxide

The third greenhouse gas of concern in this context is nitrous oxide. This is also produced by manure lagoons, but fertilisers used in crop farming also contribute to the problem. 'Aha! The vegans are damaging the planet, after all!' I might hear you exclaim. But don't rush too quickly to this conclusion. In fact, 80% of crops grown globally are used to feed livestock. Only 16% actually feeds humans, with the rest going to the production of textiles and biofuels.[20]

Of course we will never be able to get away from the fact that, as individuals, we will always be responsible for some impact on the earth, because we're members of societies which rely on industrial methods of food production, or because we use mobile phones or any given mode of transport. We can, however, think about the impact of what we're eating, and make positive changes. So let's look at how changing to a vegan diet could reduce our individual greenhouse gas emissions.

We know that animal-based foods produce around twice the amount of greenhouse emissions than plant-based foods.[21] Beef and dairy have particularly high emissions when compared with other products, particularly plant-based alternatives. Looking just at carbon dioxide, beef emits around 50kg of CO_2 per 100g of protein produced. To put this into context, the CO_2 emission from producing the same weight of nuts can be as little as 0.26kg.[22] This difference is just staggering. Dairy milk produces 3.15kg of CO_2 per litre, compared to less than 1kg for the same volume of soya milk.[23] In fact, one study has shown that the greenhouse emissions of the average vegan accounts for just 25% of that of a meat eater.[24] And when you consider that by replacing an animal-derived protein source with a plant-based one, you're having a double effect of reducing your carbon emissions and the amount of saturated fat you're consuming, it seems like a no-brainer, really.

It's not just land animal consumption that affects the levels of greenhouse gas emissions like this. The oceans are home to up to 80% of all life on earth, and absorb four times the amount of carbon dioxide as the Amazon rainforest.[25] The fishing method of bottom trawling is particularly harmful to the atmosphere, because it disturbs the sediment on the ocean floors, releasing CO_2.[26] Left alone, the sediment would store the carbon for millennia.

Deforestation and Land Clearance

Forests are really important pieces of land. They cover around one third of the earth's land area, and are home to about 80% of its terrestrial biodiversity.[27] We've already considered the effects of global warming, and forests are huge carbon stores, so removing them will have dire effects on atmospheric CO_2 levels. But it's not just the atmosphere that trees and forests are beneficial for.

Many people depend on forests because they live there, use the trees for fuel, and forage in them for food. Land clearance, as we'll learn more about later, also results in displacement of indigenous communities, because it removes their home, their source of fuel and food, forcing them to settle elsewhere. The forests are also home to animals. I'm sure we've all seen the same videos of injured orangutans, carrying their young and trying to escape the machinery that's pulling down their habitat. It is heartbreaking, and made even more devastating by the fact that it is all so avoidable. Not only are animals and humans displaced by land clearance, but destroying rich ecosystems also wipes out birds and insects. Deforestation, as we'll read more about later, also puts humans at risk of infection, because it destroys the barriers between humans and wild animals, allowing infections to pass between them. Further issues from land clearance include disruption of water cycles and soil degradation.

Much like we saw with the difference in carbon emissions between beef and dairy and their plant-based counterparts, there's also a massive difference in the land required for their production. Dairy milk requires nearly 9m² of land per litre produced, whilst soya milk takes just 0.66m² of land for the equivalent amount. And while we're thinking about soya, let's address one of the most annoying and anti-vegan myths that I've heard multiple times: does vegans' dependence on soya make us responsible for more climate change and land clearance than meat eaters? No, it does not. It is true that soya is often grown on land that was once a rainforest. However, only 6% of soya beans grown globally are used to feed humans, whilst 70–75% will go into feeds for farmed animals.[28] This means that meat eaters are indirectly consuming more soya than vegans. And we can't forget that we're adding onto this the problem of deforestation for animal feed and the gas emissions from farming the animals themselves.

While we're at it, let's clear up another myth. Grass-fed beef is often suggested as an alternative to the cruelty of industrial farming, but apart from being problematic because it couldn't possibly feed the world's population, and as such would result in a two-tier food system in which only the rich could afford to eat meat, if we did rely on grass-fed beef the amount of land that would need to be cleared to farm these cows would be unfathomable. This would lead to further issues of increased CO_2 emissions and destruction of ecosystems and biodiversity. It would be completely unsustainable. Currently, despite 26% of the earth's land surface being used for grazing animals used for meat and milk, they only provide 1% of the world's protein.[29]

Water Use

Water is an essential part of human existence. We use it for almost everything we do. But it's also a limited resource. As the climate changes, it becomes more limited, and there are vast areas on earth experiencing water scarcity. In fact, 1.42 billion people live in areas of high or extremely high water vulnerability.[30] There are many reasons why water can become scarce; sometimes demand outstrips supply, and sometimes supply dips because of reducing quantity or quality.

As the global population grows towards a predicted 10 billion people by 2050, the demand for water will only continue to rise. With 70% of all water drawn from aquifers being used for agriculture, including both crops and animals, feeding a growing population will put enormous pressure on water supplies.

We cannot ignore the fact that the production of meat also involves irrigation and growing of crops for animal feed. Beef is the worst culprit, having an environmental impact which far outweighs that of dairy, other meats and egg production. It uses twenty eight times more land and eleven times more water, and produces five times more greenhouse gas emissions than any other animal-based foods.[31] Moreover, livestock production is a really inefficient use of water (and land), because most of the energy in the plants fed to them will be wasted in the animals' metabolic processes and in the formation of non-edible tissues that never even reach the consumer's plate. The very nature of producing animal proteins, by the fact that they need to be fed crops, means that all animal-derived foods use more water than plant-based foods. Even a chicken breast, just one chicken breast, takes over 735 litres of water to produce – the same amount could fill up your bathtub nearly five times.[32] The bottom line is that producing animal protein is a really inefficient process, which could be bypassed if humans just ate the crops we fed them ourselves.

Yet there is hope! Yes, our global population is booming, and yes, we do need to be more careful with our water use to ensure fewer people experience water scarcity. But a plant-based diet could be the answer to this, as it offers a considerable water conservation benefit. The average water footprint per calorie for beef is 20 times greater than that for cereals and starchy roots,[31] whilst its water footprint for protein content is 6 times that of pulses. Milk, eggs and chicken have a footprint of around 1.5 times that of pulses. Vegetables generally have an even lower water footprint, and if all meat was replaced with the equivalent amount of crops, it would result in a reduction of food-related water footprint of around 30% for the average American citizen.[31]

Pollution

I want to consider both air and ocean pollution in this section. Let's first think about the atmosphere.

Air pollution

We've already talked about emissions and how they are harmful by causing global warming, but what about particles that are emitted which directly harm human health? We often think about pollution in terms of exhaust fumes that result in lung disease and a shortened life expectancy in those who are exposed. But did you know that agriculture directly causes pollution, not only from the transportation of food products, but through their farming and production as well?

Air pollution is one of the greatest environmental risks to health, and is estimated to have caused 4.2 million premature deaths globally in 2019.[33] These deaths occur because of cardiovascular diseases like heart disease and stroke, and respiratory disorders like chronic obstructive pulmonary disease, chest infections, and cancers. In Europe, agriculture is the single biggest cause of air pollution. It's mainly caused by nitrogen-containing compounds, like ammonia (NH_3). These usually come from heavy use of fertilisers on fields and from livestock waste, and they combine with other pollutants that come from industrial processes. This forms particulate pollutants, small particles that can enter the lungs, causing damage to tissues and affecting lung function, resulting in premature death. And once again, the farming of cattle is the leading culprit in the UK. Those poor cows. It's really not their fault, but the ammonia from cattle provides around half of all ammonia emitted.[34]

Ocean pollution

The oceans, depressingly, are full of plastic waste. It has been reported that there are now 150 million tonnes of plastic floating in the ocean, and that we add another 8 million tonnes every year.[35] Some of these plastics come from items we use every day – carrier bags, plastic bottles and disposable cutlery – but Greenpeace reports that 20% of plastic in the ocean comes from human activities at sea, mainly fishing.[36] They have previously described how 640,000 tonnes of 'ghost gear' enters the ocean every year – equivalent in weight to more than 50,000 double decker buses.[37] Ghost gear is fishing equipment that is lost or abandoned at sea, often because it is cheaper to leave it there than to haul it back to land.

It's not just the fishing industry that is adding to the already drastic plastic pollution of the oceans. We are unwittingly doing it ourselves by wearing clothing made from synthetic fabrics. Microplastics leach out of these fabrics when clothing is laundered. These then end up in the food chain when they are consumed by fish, and in humans when they eat those contaminated fish. Unfortunately, giving up fish in our diet won't completely remedy the problem, as microplastics have also been found in drinking water and can enter our food if we store and heat it in plastic containers. But at least we can reduce our exposure by eliminating one, unnecessary source: dietary fish.

The negative environmental impacts of the meat and dairy industries are now being widely recognised by global organisations. The UN has stated that there is no way to achieve the Paris Climate Agreement's targets without enormously scaling down worldwide animal agriculture,[38] and has suggested that a global move to a meat- and dairy-free diet is necessary.[39] One way in which we might be able to do this is through the EAT-Lancet diet. I'll tell you more about this in the 'Vegan for Health' chapter.

As the world opens its eyes to the benefits of a plant-based diet for climate change, veganism suddenly doesn't seem such a strange or extreme choice.

Vegan Take-Aways

Animal agriculture is the leading cause of climate change.

Only around 16% of crops grown globally are used to feed humans; most of it goes to feed animals who are being farmed for food.

Animal-based foods produce around twice the amount of greenhouse gas emissions than plant-based foods.

The UN has stated that a global shift towards a vegan diet is vital to save the world from hunger and the worst impacts of climate change.

Global warming is contributing to human disease.

Vegan foods use less land and water and emit less CO_2.

Around 26% of the earth's land surface is used for grazing animals in the meat and dairy industries, even though they only provide 1% of the world's protein sources.

3

Vegan for Health

'The human body has no more need for cows' milk than it does for dogs' milk, horses' milk, or giraffes' milk.' — Dr Michael Klaper

I hadn't initially intended for this book to be primarily about health, well at least not in the context of how becoming vegan is the best choice for our health. Although I've always accepted that a good vegan diet is probably one of the best ways of eating for health and longevity, I've always been primarily about staying well as an ethical vegan, and advocating for veganism as an acceptable choice, which need not be feared by the medical profession. But, as my years as a vegan doctor, mum and writer have gone on, I've learned so much about plant-based diets for health that I can't deny their supremacy over almost any omnivorous diet.

Veganism has previously had a mixed reputation for its effects on health, and in some ways it still does. You only have to watch an Instagram reel from a vegan physician, then another from a keto influencer to see how widely varying opinions on the same nutrition topic can be. But this is the nature of food science. Even for me as a doctor and a scientist, I can see just how conflicting and confusing the evidence is; for every paper that you find which tells you how good a vegan diet is for a particular health benefit, you'll find another paper which declares the same for keto, or low fat, or some other diet.

Yet the evidence for a healthy vegan diet is becoming stronger. An increasing number of bigger and more thorough studies are showing a clear, indisputable association between a plant-heavy diet and a reduction in the risk of disease. And it seems that we *can* conclude that a well-balanced vegan diet is very healthy indeed. In fact, the British Dietetic Association (BDA) stated that 'Plant-based diets can support healthy living at every age and life stage' – a clear affirmation that veganism really is ok, and isn't likely to kill you.[40]

This statement goes on to say, 'But as with any diet, you should plan your plant-based eating to meet your nutritional needs.' I would argue that in a world of ultra-processed, junky foods of questionable nutritional value, *everybody's* diets need to be well planned in order to provide what we need for good health. However, as vegans, our diets seem to be under much more intense scrutiny than everyone else's. Ever since I became vegan, I found this point really ironic; we're so much more likely to be thinking carefully about our nutritional intake and our health, yet everybody has something to say about just how dangerous or risky they think our lifestyle can be. It is true that as vegans, there are some nutrients that we must consider because they can be slightly more difficult to obtain without the use of animal-derived products. But that doesn't detract from the good that living vegan can do, and it is the whole point of the next section, so worry not!

The other consideration that we need to make is that not every vegan diet is equal. While a plant-based or vegan diet *can* be very healthy and help to prevent and even treat many diseases, it is important to remember that not every vegan will always eat healthily. In fact, you could call yourself a vegan, and eat plant-based nuggets, burgers and fish fingers every day, and not even sniff a whole fruit or vegetable. So you'd be doing wonders for the animals, and a little better for the planet than the average meat eater, but your body wouldn't thank you.

Although junk-food vegan diets can contain less saturated fat and more fibre than a diet rich in animal proteins, the optimal diet is one rich in whole foods, including grains, legumes, seeds, nuts, fruits and vegetables. If you are going vegan for your health, or if you are a health-conscious vegan, make sure to ditch the vegan cheese and meat replacements for whole-food sources of protein, with a whole-food plant-based (WFPB) diet. As you will gather from my recipes, I'm almost WFPB, but not 100% of the time. If even veganism seems like a daunting change from how you are living now, I can imagine that embarking upon a WFPB diet might seem like an almost impossible task, and later we will discuss how to make small changes to an overall healthier, kinder way of life.

So, what are the health benefits of adopting a vegan diet? There are so many positive effects of a vegan diet on certain chronic diseases, with such compelling evidence, that I could probably write a short book on each one, and how plant-based eating could prevent, or even reverse the disease process. Part of that will, of course be the reduction and removal of harmful animal proteins, but we're also learning so much about the benefits of plants. Fibre is just a wonder-substance. And when you add things like antioxidants and a high concentration of vitamins and minerals, you really can harness the power of plants. But, I haven't got a whole book per disease, or even a whole chapter, so I am going to squeeze as much convincing evidence into this next section as I possibly can. While it would be hard to find some aspect of human health that isn't impacted upon by good nutrition, I will only include the conditions for which we are certain that a plant-based diet is beneficial, because we have a good amount of evidence.

And all this evidence points to one conclusion: we should all consider switching to a vegan diet.

Obesity

I want to start with obesity, because it has become so common, and is implicated in so many other disease processes, that it is the one condition I think most physicians wish we could just eliminate. Attitudes about obesity are changing, albeit slowly. Not long ago, we believed that it was solely under the control of the individual. How harmful this belief was. To put all of the responsibility for what we now know is a complex, chronic disease onto the person experiencing it is so unhelpful. Cruel, even.

Defined as a body mass index (BMI) of more than $30kg/m^2$, we are now starting to understand that obesity is the result of a very complex set of conditions, including one's genetics and the switching on of those genes by an almost immeasurable number of environmental conditions. What it isn't, is due purely and simply to what a person eats. Sadly, we're also gaining an understanding that it is very difficult to treat and reverse obesity. As a clinician, I am concerned about the rise in prevalence of obesity because of its associations with heart disease, diabetes, liver and kidney disease, certain cancers, osteoarthritis and many other health conditions. There is also the fact that it is, not surprisingly, so tied into an individual's mental health, quality of life, and sense of wellbeing.

The most recent figures are shocking: in the UK, 64% of adults over 18 are living with overweight or obesity, and 26% of the population have obesity.[41] When the stark reality that over a quarter of our population have a chronic disease that can lead to cancer, cardiovascular disease and reduced quality of life, surely we need to find ways to prevent and treat this.

Anybody who has experienced difficulties with their weight will know that, while you may lose weight relatively quickly and easily with various diet plans, it is often very hard to keep the weight off. Healthcare professionals are keenly aware of this difficulty. As well as a plethora of patient stories of 'yo-yo' dieting and weight losses and gains, the evidence for different methods of weight loss often show the same thing: it's just so hard to maintain weight loss. Studies showing when diets such as very low calorie, ketogenic, or low fat are successful for weight loss, frequently demonstrate that in follow up 1 or 2 years later, weight has been regained. And often there is an even greater weight gain than before. But this is where plant-based diets for weight loss could differ.

You will probably notice a couple of recurring studies throughout this book, so let me explain why. Good data relies on good studies, and one important aspect of a good study is sample size. This is how many participants were included. Obviously, the more participants there are, the more likely it is that the results actually reflect the statistics in the real population. Another important aspect is time. A quick snapshot of a situation, whilst sometimes useful, is not as informative as a study which has followed up its participants for many years. Nutrition is very hard to study well, for reasons like how it relies on participants' memories of what they've eaten, as well as their honesty and understanding, and also because of 'confounding factors'; our lifestyle and health are impacted upon by so much more that what we eat.

Helpfully, there have been two large cohort studies that have provided some very reliable and good evidence, because they have included huge numbers of participants, and they have followed these people up over many years. These two cohorts are the Adventist

Health Studies in the USA and EPIC-Oxford in Europe. Both of these have provided a wealth of information about how we eat affects our health. And because the Adventists in America have a much higher number of vegetarians than the general public, we'll be drawing upon the results of studies based on this population a lot, as they provide so much information on the effects of meat-free diets, when compared with the meat eaters from the same demographic group.

The large population in the AHS-2 (Adventist Health Study-2), which included 96,000 participants, has shown us that the vegans in the group had, on average, a BMI of 5 points lower that non-vegetarians.[42] More studies, including EPIC-Oxford[43,44] and others[45] also back this finding up, with the EPIC-Oxford group showing that vegans gain weight more slowly than vegetarians and meat eaters. What's also useful to know is that not only do vegans have a lower BMI, but a plant-based diet seems to be useful for weight loss, too, with one meta-analysis showing that a vegan diet resulted in greater weight loss than vegetarian ones, when compared to non-vegetarian dicts.[46]

But what about maintenance? Several studies have demonstrated that a whole-food, plant-based diet can help to avoid regaining weight after losing it, as well as continued weight loss beyond just the first few months, compared with non-vegan, or other weight loss diets.[47-49]

There are lots of reasons why healthy vegan diets work for weight loss and maintenance of a healthy body weight. Firstly, plant foods are less calorie dense, meaning that for the same volume of food, plant-based will contain fewer calories than animal-based. This means that you will feel far fuller if you consume 200kcal of vegetables than you would on the same quantity of meat that provides 200kcal. Healthy vegan diets also contain less fat, which has been proven to help contribute towards weight loss. However, the magical ingredient of plant foods, that we're going to discuss again and again, is fibre. In the case of weight control, fibre works by reducing the amount of calories that your gut absorbs,[50] exerting a higher thermic effect,[51] optimising the microbiome (we'll cover this a bit more later), improving insulin levels,[52] and promoting the secretion of gut hormones which inform your brain when you are full.[53]

In reducing the effects of obesity, we can improve so many other aspects of our health. Many of these disease processes are due to inflammation, and we know that obesity is a pro-inflammatory state, with adipocytes (fat cells) releasing various hormones and chemicals, including pro-inflammatory cytokines. This is what leads to the plethora of obesity-related disease processes, many of which will be covered in this book. We are going to read about how plant-based diets can benefit these conditions not only by reducing body weight, but also by exerting effects directly on those processes, too. Let's read on to find out how.

So what do we mean when we talk about inflammation?

The word inflammation might make you think about an area of your body that you have injured, or that has become infected, and I'm guessing that when you imagine that, you think of redness, warmth or pain. You'd be quite right, in describing this condition as inflammation. But inflammation can also occur 'systemically', or throughout the body. With the injured finger or knee, the redness, warmth and pain is caused by the production of substances which are described as 'pro-inflammatory', such as oxidants and cytokines. These chemicals act as messengers to alert our immune system that it needs to get to work in that area. Everything I am describing here is a normal, healthy physiological process. An injury is often described, in medical terms, as an 'acute' problem. This describes the fact that it is short lived, having come on quickly, and will likely resolve quite rapidly, too. When the effects of an injury or disease goes on for a long time, or a disease process is of the slow-burning kind, then we call this 'chronic'.

Chronic inflammation is the persistent overproduction of these pro-inflammatory agents, substances like cytokines, oxidants and chemokines. This is where inflammation turns from physiological to pathological, and leads to various diseases and chronic conditions, such as heart disease, diabetes and cancers, because of damage to tissues, infiltration of inflammatory cells and an exaggerated immune response. Whilst inflammation around an injury has a clear mechanism, and the purpose is quite obvious, it's hard to rationalise the chronic inflammation that occurs due to what we're eating and how we're living. It doesn't really have a purpose, but it leads to so many harmful processes. This is why we need to consider how to prevent ending up in a pro-inflammatory state. And amongst other ways, diet is one change we can make to reduce inflammatory responses within our bodies.

In fact, you may even have heard about an 'anti-inflammatory diet'. The truth is, however, that there isn't just one anti-inflammatory diet, but there are foods and dietary patterns that are beneficial in reducing inflammation and reducing the risk of inflammatory diseases. The most popular and well-known anti-inflammatory diet is the Mediterranean Diet. This was designed by scientists in the 1970s, and was based on the eating patterns of people who live around the Mediterranean. It focuses on unprocessed plant foods, but does allow for a moderate amount of fish, meat and dairy. The benefits, however, come primarily from the plant part. It is rich in antioxidants, fibre, vitamins and minerals.

What an anti-inflammatory diet should do, is remove the elements that promote inflammation, like refined carbohydrates, saturated fat, salt, added sugar and alcohol, and be rich in anti-inflammatory foods like fruits, vegetables, nuts, seeds and legumes.

I just want to make a short comment on fish as part of an anti-inflammatory diet. Oily fish is incorporated into the Mediterranean Diet, and this is because of its omega-3 fatty acid content, which is known to be anti-inflammatory and protective of some inflammatory conditions. However, in the 21st century, eating fish also comes with risks, including its microplastics content, and exposure to heavy metals. And don't forget that this book is the complete guide to living more kindly; omega-3 can be taken as a supplement sourced from algae, removing the need to take fish from already depleted oceans, and force them to endure unpleasant deaths.

Type 2 Diabetes Mellitus

Type 2 Diabetes Mellitus (T2DM) is a very common but serious condition, with 3.8 million people in the UK experiencing it, and 5 million people being at risk of developing it.[54] T2DM is a chronic disease in which our tissues become resistant to the effects of insulin. Let me explain a little more. Insulin is a hormone which is released after eating, and is responsible for moving the sugars we have eaten and absorbed, from our bloodstream into our cells to be used as energy for normal cellular processes. If the sugar can't be moved into the cells, it stays in the blood causing a rise in blood sugar levels. When these rises in blood sugar are persistent and chronic it can be harmful to our bodies, and in the long term causes damage to organs, including kidneys, nerves, eyes and the cardiovascular system. It can also lead to death; in 2019 type 2 diabetes caused 1.5 million deaths worldwide.[55]

Insulin resistance is a consequence of storing too much fat in the liver and muscles. This is usually because of diet, and therefore can be prevented and even reversed. Whilst insulin resistance can occur by itself, it is usually a precursor to type 2 diabetes, and it isn't unusual for somebody to be diagnosed as 'pre-diabetic' before receiving a diagnosis of diabetes. By avoiding the storage of excess fats in our organs, we can potentially avoid insulin resistance and T2DM. Associations have been made between T2DM and diets high in animal proteins; in one study, every 20g increase in animal protein intake was associated with a 7% increased risk of type 2 diabetes.[56] But the good news is that this is reversible; this same study also demonstrated that for every 20g of animal protein that was replaced with plants, the risk of T2DM fell by 20%.

It has long been understood that vegetarians and vegans have a lower risk of T2DM.[57-59] We have already discussed that this will be, in part, due to the reduced risk of obesity and the removal of the direct effect of animal proteins and saturated fat, but we also know that fibre improves postprandial blood sugar and insulin levels. Didn't I tell you that fibre would keep coming up as a wonder-substance? A healthy vegan diet has a high fibre content, as well as the added goodness of plant-derived compounds such as antioxidants like polyphenols, and polyunsaturated fatty acids (PUFAs), which can activate anti-inflammatory pathways.

But what has inflammation got to do with T2DM? I've just told you all about how diabetes is caused by excess fat storage, and high blood sugars, but inflammation really does play a part. Not just in the development of T2DM, but inflammation also becomes a result of the condition, meaning that people with diabetes tend to end up in a bit of a vicious circle. Research seems to show that low-grade inflammation is associated with the risk of developing T2DM by causing insulin resistance,[60] but then the resulting high blood sugar levels increases the production of pro-inflammatory proteins and cytokines.[61]

Whole-food plant-based diets often contain foods which have a lower glycaemic index (GI), which has a beneficial effect on blood sugars. Glycaemic index is the way of describing the extent to which a food alters your blood sugar. Foods with a low GI have the least impact, causing just a small rise in blood sugar, and those with a high GI cause blood sugars to rise more rapidly and to a higher level. While we are discussing blood sugar levels, I want to address a trend that I have noticed over the last couple of years. There seems to be a subset of social media doctors and health influencers who are obsessed with blood sugars, who have tried to convince their followers that blood sugars shouldn't be rising at all. A variation in blood sugar level is normal after eating. Of course, eating healthful whole-foods which offer multiple benefits, as well as being an energy source, is the most ideal way to eat, rather than consuming lots of highly processed, high sugar foods with little fibre or other nutrients. Concentrating on eating like this, rather than becoming obsessed with what our blood sugars are doing when we aren't diabetic, is likely to be more helpful in staying well. Lastly, specific micronutrients like magnesium are also found in higher concentrations in plant-based diets, and this has also been associated with improved glucose metabolism.[62]

Not only do we know that vegans will be at reduced risk of diabetes, but we can also be quite confident that we could prescribe plant-based diets for the prevention of those who are already at increased risk, because as we've already read, a plant-based diet improves insulin resistance.[63] Even small amounts of red meat and poultry seem to disproportionately increase a person's risk of T2DM.[60] Considering how closely associated diet and the risk of diabetes is, it's really no big surprise that plant-based diets could also be useful in treating diabetes in those already diagnosed,[64,65] and in reducing the harmful effects of T2DM.[66]

Reducing the ill effects of insulin resistance has implications beyond diabetes too: insulin resistance is a predictor of heart disease risk.[67] Ischaemic heart disease (IHD) is yet another serious condition which can be prevented and even treated with a healthy vegan diet. Read on to find out how.

Metabolic Syndrome

Metabolic syndrome describes a condition where three or more of the following risk factors are present: central obesity, raised blood triglyceride levels, low HDL levels, raised blood pressure, or raised fasting blood sugar levels. Metabolic syndrome increases the risk of cardiovascular diseases, like ischaemic heart disease, and the primary underlying mechanism is insulin resistance.

As we will discuss elsewhere, we know that plant-based diets are associated with a lower risk of most of these, and as such a vegan diet can be a way of managing or preventing metabolic syndrome.[68] This is down to several mechanisms, from the reduced energy intake, higher intake of polyphenols

*and other antioxidants, improved insulin resistance, and re-
duced intake of saturated fatty acids and haem iron. In fact,
red meat has been associated with metabolic syndrome,[69]
while vegan diets seem to be preventative [70].*

Cardiovascular Disease

Heart disease, sometimes called ischaemic heart disease (IHD) or
coronary heart disease (CHD), is caused by a build-up of cholesterol
in the small blood vessels that supply the muscle walls of the heart.
These vessels then either become narrowed or blocked by this build
up, known as atheroma, or the plaque formed by the cholesterol can
rupture. This then causes a blood clot to form, which occludes the
vessel completely, causing a heart attack, or in medical terms, a myocardial infarction (MI). This can happen slowly over a long time,
and a person with IHD might experience angina – usually a central
or left-sided chest pain that occurs on exertion, and is relieved by
rest – but when the vessel is fully occluded, the area of heart muscle
it supplies doesn't receive sufficient oxygen and becomes damaged,
or even dies, causing severe chest pain, collapse, nausea, clamminess,
and even death.

If a heart attack is survived, it can lead to heart failure, a condition
where the heart muscle has become damaged and doesn't pump
blood around the body as effectively as it should. The term *cardiovascular disease* refers to this mechanism throughout the blood vessels of the entire body. So whilst we're mostly talking about heart
disease in this section, the blood vessels of any part of the body can
become blocked in the same way, risking blood supply to the body
part that the blood vessel supplies, and it's usually due to the same
mechanisms. Therefore, removing and reducing the risk factors for

IHD can also reduce the risk of disease of other parts of the cardiovascular system.

It all sounds rather gloomy and serious, doesn't it? Well, of course experiencing IHD is unpleasant, frightening, and can have a huge impact on your health. But so many cases of heart disease are preventable. In fact, it is thought that around 80% of cardiovascular disease could be prevented with diet, exercise and avoidance of smoking.[71] It is well understood by clinicians that atherosclerosis, the mechanism by which the blood vessels become narrowed in IHD, is caused primarily by LDL-C (low density lipoprotein cholesterol), sometimes known as the 'bad cholesterol'.[72]

Studies have shown that vegan diets are associated with lower blood LDL-C levels.[73,74] Firstly, cholesterol is found only in animal-derived foods, so it makes sense that by following a vegan diet, by its very nature free of dietary cholesterol, rather than one rich in animal proteins, one should be at lower risk of IHD.

Secondly, we know that saturated fat in the diet increases LDL-C levels, and a vegan diet tends to have a lower saturated fat content. Yes, meat, especially red meat, contains far more saturated fat than plant-based foods, but that doesn't mean that a vegan diet contains none. There are two exceptions to the rule that vegan food is low in saturated fat: both palm fat and coconut oil have a high saturated fat content, and should be consumed in moderation, if at all.

It is for these reasons that a vegan diet can reduce the risk of heart disease and death from IHD.[75] Do you recall those two studies with huge cohorts in the US and Europe? Well, they are relevant here, too. The Adventist Health Study-2 showed a 19% reduced risk of IHD in vegetarians,[76] while the EPIC-Oxford study found that the risk of hospitalisation and death from IHD was 32% lower in a similar group.[77]

It does seem that plant-based diets are largely beneficial for cardiovascular health, and it's not just about what you *don't* eat. Let me tell you, briefly, about dietary cholesterol: cholesterol is an organic compound which is important in the human body for lots of different processes, including making vitamin D and some hormones. Every cell in our body can make cholesterol when it is required, although they can't break it down.[78] What our bodies can do, instead, to get rid of excess cholesterol is to excrete it in the bowel, in bile. So whilst it makes sense that eating less dietary cholesterol will result in lower blood cholesterol levels, we can also influence those levels by consuming more foods that block cholesterol absorption in the bowel, or increase the amount we excrete. And guess what? It's really no surprise that these foods are all plant-based.

Phytosterols are components of plant cell membranes, similar in structure to cholesterol. It has been known for a long time that phytosterols block cholesterol absorption, with a higher intake being associated with lower LDL-C levels.[79] You have probably seen these sterols and stanols advertised to you in products that are marketed to help to bring your cholesterol level down. Products like 'Benecol' and 'Flora Pro-Activ' are sold with a promise to treat your high cholesterol, but what these companies don't tell you is that many plant-based foods naturally contain phytosterols, albeit in lower concentrations. To increase your intake, make sure to include plenty of beans, lentils, nuts and seeds, but the evidence does show that there is further benefit from adding phytosterol-fortified foods to our diets if there is a diagnosis of high cholesterol, as it is hard to eat the amount required to really impact high levels.

Fibre makes another appearance as a wonder-food, this time implicated in cholesterol metabolism. Fibre, amongst all of its other amazing properties, helps to reduce blood cholesterol levels. This is by both decreasing the absorption of dietary fats in the gut but also increasing the amount of cholesterol excreted in the stools in bile.[80] One meta-analysis of the evidence for the benefit of fibre in cardiovascular disease demonstrated that people who consume the highest amounts of dietary fibre reduce their chances of developing IHD and stroke by somewhere between 7% and 24%. Another study found that the risk of coronary events was 14% lower for each extra 10g per day of fibre consumed, and the risk of coronary death was 27% lower.[81] But it's not just the effects of fibre on the absorption and excretion of cholesterol that makes plant-based foods healthier for our hearts. Fibre is implicated in the health of the gut microbiome, which itself can produce beneficial substances, like the short-chain fatty acid (SCFA), butyrate, that influence our cardiovascular health. But how?

We know that ischaemic heart disease is, in part, driven by inflammation. Although the coronary arteries are being blocked by fatty deposits, inflammatory processes are involved in this laying down of lipids and cells. For this reason, IHD is now recognised as an inflammatory condition. Associations have been made between markers of inflammation in the body and the risk of developing heart disease; one study demonstrated that a high blood level of a commonly tested inflammatory marker, CRP (C-reactive protein), was a predictor for developing IHD.[82] The gut microbiome is implicated in this relationship between inflammation and heart disease because a reduced fibre intake could result in changes to the bacteria which then produce less butyrate, leading to localised gut wall inflammation, allowing bacterial toxins that cause IHD to leak through into the bloodstream.[83] It has been demonstrated that when compared with the American Heart Association-recommended diet for people with established heart disease, a vegan diet can have a greater effect of reducing inflammatory markers.[84]

Another way in which the microbiome impacts on heart disease is through some of the products of digestion of meat. When bacteria break down and ferment the foods we eat, they produce multiple chemicals and substances, like the butyrate we were just considering. Some of these can be harmful, moreso if it is animal proteins which the bacteria are metabolising. The Western diet, being rich in meat, promotes bacterial production of TMA (trimethylamine), which the liver changes into TMAO (trimethylamine N-oxide), which is known to contribute to the process of atherosclerosis[85]. A vegan diet is lower in TMAO because of the absence of meat. The fact that a vegan diet will have a higher content of antioxidants from all of the fruits and vegetables has also been associated with reduced mortality from cardiovascular disease.

So what about treating heart disease? Is it possible to treat IHD and blocked arteries with a WFPB diet? If you recall, the mechanism of cardiovascular disease is a blocking up of the blood vessels with fatty deposits. There are several ways in which heart disease is treated conventionally, using medications and/or surgical interventions, but to actually clear a vessel of its blockage, it's usually a surgical intervention that is used. This can involve either stretching the remaining bit of open lumen with a balloon and popping a stent in there to keep the vessel open, or completely bypassing the vessel with a new one, usually taken from a patient's own leg. It seems unlikely that a dietary intervention could clear significant blockage from a blood vessel. However there is evidence that, under strict controls, this is possible.[86,87] The studies in which the blockage of coronary arteries was reversed with a plant-based diet involved small numbers of participants. Although it would be difficult to recruit enough people to really increase the power of these studies, because the dietary changes that led to the reversal of the blocked arteries were very strict indeed, I'm hopeful that there is a role for a WFPB diet in the treatment of heart disease. Nevertheless, the evidence for its role in the *prevention* of heart disease is strong.

Hypertension

Hypertension, or raised blood pressure, is a concern because it is associated with not just cardiovascular disease, but also kidney disease and dementia. Blood pressure is, as the name suggests, the pressure that the blood in your veins and arteries exerts on the walls of these blood vessels. A diagnosis of hypertension is made when your blood pressure reading is 140/90mmHg or higher when you are in clinic, or an average reading of 135/85mmHg or greater when at home. It is quite normal for your blood pressure to fluctuate, but we worry when those fluctuations regularly go too high, or when the baseline is persistently raised. This is because increased blood pressure damages what we call 'end organs', which are the organs last to be affected in a disease process. So, for example, raised blood pressure can cause chronic kidney disease by damaging the renal system, and strokes by damaging the vessels to the brain.

One thing that I always try to get patients with hypertension to hold onto, is the fact that it is very often a reversible disease. While its effects can be catastrophic, it is possible to return your blood pressure to normal, although it can take a little bit of work. Amongst various ways of doing this, you can increase your activity levels, reduce your salt and alcohol intake, and of course change your diet. It has been demonstrated that those who follow a plant-based diet tend to have lower blood pressure,[91,92] and we know that diets rich in animal proteins are associated with hypertension.[93] It is a healthy vegan diet's propensity for being low in saturated fat and salt, which we know can lead to hypertension, that makes it useful in preventing a raised blood pressure. But we also know that it is possible to actually treat and reverse hypertension with a vegan diet to reduce high blood pressure after diagnosis.[94] As well as a lower salt intake and a reduction in inflammation, there is also evidence that the higher vitamin C and polyphenol content of plant-based diets can contribute to the mechanism of lowering of blood pressure.[95]

So it probably isn't any coincidence that a diet which was specifically developed for the management of hypertension, is based largely on a whole-food plant-based diet. While the DASH (Dietary Approaches to Stop Hypertension) diet isn't solely plant-based, it does emphasise fruits, vegetables, wholegrains, nuts and legumes, and while it does include low-fat dairy, it limits total and saturated fat, cholesterol, red and processed meats, sweets, added sugars, and sugary drinks.[96] It has been shown to reduce blood pressure, alongside other lifestyle changes, such as weight loss, exercise and reducing salt intake, and has even shown a positive effect on blood pressure without the use of medication.[97] The DASH diet has also been shown to reduce LDL-C,[98] and to reduce the risk of diabetes,[99] and death from cardiovascular disease.[100] This is probably due to same effects that we read about in the above sections for ischaemic heart disease and diabetes, where a plant-based diet removed harmful saturated fat and cholesterol intake, but added all the goodness of fibre, antioxidants and more.

Microplastics and Health

Why are we so concerned with the discovery of microplastics being just about everywhere? Well, it seems that plastics aren't very good for our health, and could even be rather detrimental. Plastics contain more than 10,000 chemicals, some of which are known to be carcinogenic, and others are known to disrupt human hormone production.[88] They've also been described as capable of increasing the risk for premature births, neurodevelopmental disorders, male reproductive birth defects, infertility, obesity, cardiovascular disease and renal disease.[89] A recent study in the New England Journal of Medicine found some of these microplastics inside the atheromatous plaques removed from the carotid arteries of patients with cardiovascular disease.[90] As I explained earlier in this chapter, an atheromatous plaque is what blocks blood vessels in people with cardiovascular disease, and it is made from fatty deposits and white blood cells. This study found that these plaques contain microplastics in 58% of participants, which were likely consumed through their diets. But why does this matter? Because the study also found that those who did have these microplastics present were more likely to die or go on to have a heart attack or stroke than those who didn't have them.

Cancers

Several cancers have been associated with a diet heavy in meat and animal products, with an increased risk of bowel, breast, lung, endometrial and liver cancers seen in those who eat a higher intake of red meat.[101,102] The most commonly discussed and known about, however, is colorectal cancer, where the connection is indisputable.[103] Let's have a look at how animal protein-rich diets have been associated with some types of cancer.

Colorectal cancer

Colorectal cancer is the fourth most common cancer in the UK, with around 120 people being diagnosed every day.[104] It is also sometimes called bowel cancer, but the term colorectal includes cancers that can occur anywhere in the large bowel, also known as the colon, or the rectum. Evidence shows that processed meat like sausages, bacon and ham are the worst culprits for being associated with colorectal cancer, being classified as a group 1 carcinogen.[105] To put this into context, cigarettes are also in this group, meaning the evidence shows that these substances *do* cause cancer. It's not very often that scientists can say with such certainty that something is 'causative', but the evidence that processed red meat causes bowel cancer is very strong. Other red meats aren't far behind, and are in group 2, i.e. they are *likely* to cause cancer, and Cancer Research UK estimates that 13% of colorectal cancer cases in the UK are caused by eating red and processed meats.[104]

The effect is dose-dependent, too; the International Agency for Research on Cancer (IARC) working group estimated that for every additional 100 g of red meat eaten, the risk of colorectal cancer increases by about 18%.[105] As such, recommendations have been made that red meat intake should be limited, and processed red meats should be avoided.[106] I'm still fascinated by the fact that processed red meats and cigarettes are treated so differently by UK doctors, however. Whilst you would be certain that you would be on the receiving end of education and support to stop if you told your GP you smoked cigarettes, can we say that we would receive the same treatment if we disclosed that we ate processed and red meat? Obviously, my patients do. I'm always honest about the effects of consuming red and processed meat, and I inform my patients that the evidence shows that processed meat, in particular, is harmful to human health, and should not be consumed. I think that not only do

most GPs *not* do the same, but many will still be eating these products themselves. This is amazing, really. Could you imagine knowing
that most GPs probably smoke cigarettes?

There are several mechanisms by which red and processed meats
cause an increased risk of colorectal cancer. Firstly, when cooked,
meat produces harmful substances. The main culprits are haem,[107]
N-nitroso compounds (NOCs),[108] and heterocyclic amines
(HCAs).[108] Haem is a ring-shaped, iron-containing molecule, found
in haemoglobin, the protein in blood that transports oxygen around
the body. As such, it's only found in animal proteins, thus vegans
manage to avoid it entirely. This is good news when we know its effects on the bowel wall are implicated in the development of colorectal cancer. N-nitroso compounds result from nitrites and nitrates,
additives used in some meats as preservatives. They are known to
be carcinogenic, and to make matters worse, the natural production
of NOCs by the cells in our bowel wall is further stimulated by the
presence of haem from meat.[110] As exogenous (originating outside
of the body) NOCs are formed from the consumption of processed
meats, again, they are entirely avoided by vegans. Finally, HCAs are
chemical compounds produced by cooking meat, and some are mu-
tagenic, meaning they can alter genes, which results in cancer.

As with all of the elements of risk reduction with a vegan diet
that have been discussed so far, it isn't merely the removal of these
harmful substances that help to prevent colorectal cancer in vegans,
but benefit is gained from what can be added to the diet. Again, I
can't understate the benefits of the inclusion of more fibre in our diets. It has been demonstrated that diets with a higher fibre content
result in a reduced risk of colorectal cancer,[111] and that doubling fibre intake could reduce the risk of colorectal cancer by up to 40%.[112]
It is thought that the effects that fibre exert on the intestine – increasing stool bulk, diluting carcinogens in the stool, and reducing

the amount of time that faeces remain in contact with the walls of the large intestine – all contribute towards this reduced risk.

Once again, we can't ignore all the vitamins, minerals and antioxidants that come with fibre-rich foods, and the effect of fibre on the gut microbiome. Those who take a high-fibre diet, like healthy vegans, have gut bacteria which produce more SCFAs, such as butyrate, which are protective against colorectal cancer[113]. Conversely, it is also understood that in the guts of people who eat a lot of meat, the microbiome produces substances associated with an increased risk of colorectal cancer. Finally, the high fat intake associated with animal-based diets is also implicated in the increased risk of colorectal cancer.[114] This is probably due to the increased level of bile acids required in the intestine to break down these fats, which can be metabolised by the bacteria in the gut to harmful substances like deoxycholic acid, which are thought to promote colorectal cancers.[115]

The Microbiome

The word microbiome describes a community of microorganisms, including bacteria, living in any given habitat. We have these communities all over and throughout our bodies, being colonised by all kinds of bugs, and it is thought that there are roughly the same number of bacteria in the human body as there are our own cells.[116] Although there are various microbiomes throughout our anatomy, the one which I am referring to when I discuss microbiome in this book, is that of the gut.

The gut microbiota, the specific combination of microorganisms living in that particular microbiome, is more, however, than just a community of bacteria. It is, rather, part of a wider communication and signalling system, called the gut-brain axis. This system includes the central nervous system, nerves between the brain and gut, the microbiota itself, and hormones released from various glands, including in the gut and the pituitary gland.

The make-up of the gut microbiota varies depending on many different factors. The most obvious of these is what we eat, but the constitution of our microbiota develops and then changes depending on things like what kind of delivery we were born via, whether we were breast(/chest)fed as an infant, our activity levels, age, medications, and hormones. Whilst an imbalance in our microbiota, or 'dysbiosis', can lead to illness, being unwell or certain disease processes can also change our microbiota profile. One important marker of a healthy microbiome is the diversity of the bacteria within it. Plant-based diets are known to increase the diversity of gut microbes, while diets rich in animal products tend to reduce it.[117]

The balance of the types of bacteria is also really important; diets which weigh heavily towards being plant-based or vegan tend to increase the number of 'good' bacteria, which metabolise dietary fibre into healthy short-chain fatty acids, such as butyrate, acetate and proprionate. These are associated with a reduced risk of many diseases, in part because they help to reduce inflammation. When the microbiota becomes dysbiotic, there is a reduction in the amount of short-chain fatty acids (SCFAs) produced by bacteria in the gut, which compromises the integrity of the barrier formed by the gut wall. This means that inflammation can ensue, and the imbalance can lead to many chronic health disorders.

Lung cancers

Despite us knowing that 80–90% of lung cancers are attributable to tobacco,[118] associations have been made with diet, and in particular, with poor quality diets. Red meat seems to increase the risk of lung cancer, with the effect being dose-dependent: for every 120g of red meat consumed per day, the risk of lung cancer increases by 35%.[119] Once again, the mechanism points, in part, towards haem iron.[120] As we know from the colorectal cancer section above, meat contains carcinogens like haem iron, and it has been demonstrated that lung cancer cells show a greater uptake of haem than healthy lung cells.[121] It is possible that consuming carcinogens can result in harmful by-products reaching the lungs in the bloodstream. In contrast, some studies have shown that in those who have good quality diets, the risk of lung cancer is reduced,[122,123] with one meta-analysis suggesting that in those who consume a higher quantity of fruits and vegetables, the risk of lung cancer could be reduced by as much as 18%.[124] There is evidence that the healthy substances found in plant foods, like antioxidants, can mop up the harmful free radicals generated by smoking cigarettes, potentially protecting the lungs of smokers.[125] This is why a diet high in fruits, vegetables and whole grains, and low in red meat, high fat and refined foods could protect from lung cancer.

Prostate cancer

The prostate gland is found in males and people assigned male at birth and is responsible for producing the liquid part of semen. It is a walnut-sized gland that sits in the pelvis, just below the bladder. The urethra, the tube through which urine flows, passes through it. It is very common for the prostate to become enlarged as a person gets older, causing symptoms of slow urinary stream, difficulty fully emptying the bladder, and nocturia, or getting up at night to urinate frequently. In some people, these symptoms can be due to cancer in the prostate gland, which is the second most common cancer in men.

Whilst the cause of prostate cancer isn't fully understood, associations have been made with increasing age, ethnicity, height, obesity and diet.[126] Of course, these last two are of interest to us, when we are discussing the potentially protective effects of a plant-based diet, particularly when we've already discussed how obesity can be prevented and treated with a healthy vegan diet. So, it would stand to reason that being vegan and the likely resultant healthy BMI might go some way towards lowering your risk of prostate cancer.

There are many other considerations, like the potentially protective effects of an anti-inflammatory diet high in antioxidants, and the avoidance of harmful components that we already know about, like carcinogens and saturated fats. Some studies have indicated that too many saturated fats in the diet could contribute to the progression of prostate cancer because of their inflammatory properties, as well as their association with derangement of sex hormones and growth factors.[127] There is also evidence that higher cholesterol levels could be associated with an increased risk of prostate cancer,[128] and as we know, diets rich in animal products are associated with increased blood cholesterol levels.

As with colorectal cancer, HCAs from cooked meats also play a part in prostate cancer, and several studies have shown that it seems to be cooking meat very well which increases the risk.[129-131] Dairy has been implicated too; some studies show that the risk of prostate cancer is increased in people who have a high intake of diary,[132,133] as well as milk being associated with an increased risk of recurrence[134] and progression[135] in those already diagnosed. What isn't clear, however, is how this risk correlates with the type of dairy being consumed, with some of these studies making the association with high-fat milk only, while others demonstrate that it is just milk and not other dairy products. One large study that we've already discussed, the EPIC-Oxford, suggested that it is only the calcium and protein derived from dairy that are positively associated with a higher risk of prostate cancer.[136] Either way, it appears that avoiding dairy's saturated fat content as well as some cancer-associated hormones, like IGF-1,[137] could reduce the risk of experiencing prostate cancer, and that plant-based diets could be protective.[138-140]

Breast cancer

Breast cancer is the most common cancer in the UK, with almost 57,000 new cases per year.[141] Interestingly, almost one quarter of cases are associated with modifiable risk factors; 15% are linked to alcohol, hormone replacement therapy (HRT) use, or not having breast(/chest)fed an infant, and 8% are associated with obesity. Therefore, because of its beneficial effects on body weight, a plant-based diet could have a role in preventing some cases of breast cancer. But even aside from a vegan diet's positive effects on body weight, there does seem to be a specific association between animal products and breast cancer. What is more striking from the evidence, however, are the protective effects of some plant-based foods in preventing recurrence in those already diagnosed. Let's take a look at some of this evidence.

Firstly, there is a suggestion that a diet high in meat is associated with an increased risk of breast cancer,[142,143] and there are a couple of ways in which this mechanism might occur. Heterocyclic amines (HCAs) crop up again; it seems to be cooked meat in particular that has been demonstrated to have this association with breast cancer, and we know that it is the cooking of meat that produces these carcinogenic substances.[144] Associations have also been made between blood levels of total cholesterol and breast cancer,[145] and as we've already read, cholesterol tends to be higher in those who eat animal products. Saturated fat continues to be problematic with associations being made between it and certain types of breast cancers.[146] Diets high in animal products also tend to be higher in the hormone IGF-I,[147] which has been linked with several cancers, including prostate, which we learned about earlier, and breast cancer.[148]

The effects of dairy on the risk of breast cancer remain somewhat controversial. There are studies showing an association with increased risk, but also demonstrated has been a *reduction* in risk. It has been proposed that this conflict in the evidence could be due to the varying susceptibility to breast cancer at different points throughout one's life. But what does seem to be demonstrated in the studies is that replacing full fat dairy milk with soya milk could reduce the risk of breast cancer,[149] and consuming more soya, generally, could reduce the risk of recurrence and death in those who are already diagnosed.[150] This is likely because of isoflavones found in soya, which are phytoestrogens. *Oestrogen* is the hormone which is responsible for female sexual characteristics, and around 80% of breast cancers are oestrogen receptor positive (ER+).[151] This means that the breast cancer cells have oestrogen receptors on them, which can affect the treatment you might receive, but it also means that you probably won't be able to take HRT if you have a diagnosis of ER+ breast cancer. It is for this reason that for some time, the fact that there were oestrogen-like substances, *phytoestrogens*, in plant foods like soya caused a bit of a scare. However, whilst isoflavones do bind to oestrogen receptors, they are tissue selective, binding to a sub-type of receptor called beta oestrogen receptors over alpha receptors, and thus have a protective effect, in terms of breast cancer, and can help manage menopause symptoms,[152] which we'll discuss in more detail a little later.

Finally, we're back to our old friend fibre: another element of a healthy vegan diet which is implicated in the risk of developing breast cancers, and, like soya, which itself is a great source of the stuff, seems to be protective.[153] As with some of the other diseases we have been reading about, the benefit of fibre seems to be dose-dependent here too, with some studies showing that a 10g per day increase in fibre intake could be associated with a 7% risk reduction,[154] and a 20g per day increase resulting in a 15% lower risk, partly because of its effects on blood sugars, insulin levels and insulin-like growth factors, which are all associated with breast cancer. Fibre also seems to exert its effects through increasing the amount of oestrogen excreted in stools, reducing the amount circulating in the bloodstream, as well as directly inhibiting tumour growth.[155] As the evidence keeps showing us, plants are best, and you just can't get enough!

Liver cancer

It is important to know that liver cancer, when it isn't secondary to a primary cancer elsewhere in the body, is often a progression from chronic liver disease, one cause of which is metabolic dysfunction-associated steatotic liver disease (MASLD). I will tell you more about MASLD in the gastrointestinal diseases section, but, briefly, it is the disease caused by storage of too much fat in the liver, and most often this is associated with obesity. As we know, obesity is less common in vegans, and so we can assume that a healthy vegan diet could go some way towards helping to reduce the risk of liver cancers. And the evidence does seem to show that diets with lower intakes of red and processed meats are associated with a reduced risk of MASLD and therefore liver cancer.[156]

Gastrointestinal Diseases

Inflammatory bowel disease

Inflammatory bowel disease (IBD) includes both Crohn's disease (CD) and ulcerative colitis (UC). As the name suggests, they are chronic, inflammatory conditions, whose cause is unknown. Whilst UC only causes inflammation in the large bowel, CD can affect the gut anywhere from the mouth to the back passage. Symptoms of IBD can include diarrhoea, blood or mucus in the stools, abdominal pains, and weight loss. The severity of IBD can vary, and in some people it can be very debilitating. Treatments vary from medications that reduce inflammation, like steroids and aminosalicylates, to immune system modulators and biologics. These medications in themselves can be difficult to take, sometimes with quite serious side effects. Some people who have serious complications, or whose symptoms don't respond to medical treatment might even end up requiring surgery for IBD. This is usually to remove a portion of the bowel, called a resection, and it can sometimes result in them requiring a stoma.

Diet doesn't always come into the consideration of doctors treating patients with IBD, which seems just unfathomable to me. Apart from the fact that gastroenterologists look after people with this condition, literally doctors of the gut, it would also make sense that when the main purpose of an organ is to process food and extract nutrition, that when that organ is diseased, we should be looking very carefully at what foods are being put into it. Apart from a mention of specialist nutritional supplementation in special circumstances, I couldn't see much about diet in the NHS guidelines for managing IBD.[157] In a patient information leaflet from Crohn's and Colitis UK, fibre does get a mention, where they state that intake needs to be reduced during a flare-up, but that intake should be increased when a person is symptom free, as it helps to keep the bowel healthy.[158] The leaflet also mentions that some people find dairy causes flare-ups, but that there isn't much evidence for this currently. So, what is the evidence? Can a plant-based diet help with IBD?

Although we don't know what causes IBD, we do know that environmental factors play a large part, which includes diet. It is thought that a Western diet is the trigger, because in some countries, an increase in the incidence of IBD has been observed to coincide with westernisation of the diet.[159] We already know that a diet high in meat and dairy is pro-inflammatory, so it makes sense that high dietary intakes of total fats and meat have been associated with increased risk of inflammatory bowel disease.[160] Once again, fibre plays a big part; higher intake of fibre and fruits has been linked to a reduced risk of IBD,[161] and so plant-rich diets could be recommended as one component of the treatment of IBD.[162]

As we've already read earlier in this chapter, we know that the gut bacteria of those who eat mostly plants break down food to produce more SCFAs like butyrate, which is used as an energy source by the cells that line the large intestine. Another role that butyrate has is to maintain the barrier in the gut to prevent harmful substances getting through. When this barrier breaks down, the gut can become 'leaky' allowing pathogens to enter deeper layers of the gut lining or the bloodstream. This is thought to be, in part, one mechanism by which IBD can develop.[163] So, eating as many healthful foods that promote the types of bacteria which produce these protective SCFAs is likely to offer some benefit in reducing the risk of IBD and its complications. And these foods are mostly plants.

This does beg the question: why aren't UK gastroenterologists recommending a plant-based diet for patients with inflammatory bowel disease? Well, it isn't entirely true that they aren't; there are doctors in the UK, usually part of the membership of Plant-Based Health Professionals UK, who advocate for a healthy vegan diet for all kinds of chronic diseases. Dr Alan Desmond is a gastroenterologist who is passionate about prescribing plants to his patients, and that's because he's read the evidence. Do look him up, if you haven't already, particularly if you have any gastrointestinal disorders and want to know more about how plant-based eating can impact this. I'll pop the details for his book in the resources section. But how do we get all doctors to read the evidence? When the cost of treating IBD can be over £10k per patient, per year,[164] it would be in the interest of the NHS to educate its clinicians on the benefits of using diet in the management of the disease.

As well as managing the symptoms and complications of inflammation in the bowel, diet could also be important in preventing the increased risk of bowel cancer that IBD poses in some people.[165] Perhaps when we know that a plant-based diet can significantly reduce our risk of colorectal cancer, ensuring that people with IBD avoid meat and take a high-fibre diet may mitigate at least some of that risk.

I do have a couple of words of warning, though. Firstly, people with inflammatory bowel disease are at higher risk of osteoporosis.[166] We'll get onto bone health a little later in this chapter, but vegans with IBD will need to manage their calcium and vitamin D intake with a little more care than those who don't have the condition. This applies to other micronutrients too, actually, as deficiencies can sometimes be seen in those with IBD, so I would consider taking supplements alongside a healthy vegan diet. However, these details need to be discussed with your gastroenterologist and dietician. Lastly, a low-fibre diet might also be necessary during flare-ups, so being vegan would mean a little more consideration of your diet during these episodes and, again, should be discussed with your specialist.

Diverticular disease

Diverticular disease is a condition which is characterised by flare-ups of abdominal pain, loose stools, possibly with bleeding, and fever. Diverticula are little out-pouches of the bowel wall caused, primarily, by the Western diet, which is lower in fibre and higher in meat and saturated fat.[167] The diverticula can be present with no symptoms, which is known as diverticulosis, and can then be called diverticular disease once symptoms occur. If these pouches become inflamed or infected, the condition is called diverticulitis. In the EPIC-Oxford study, the risk of diverticular disease was 27% lower in vegetarians, and 72% lower in vegans than in meat eaters.[45]

Because many of the risk factors for diverticulitis are the same as that for cardiovascular disease and type 2 diabetes (low-fibre diet, high red meat consumption, obesity and smoking), as well as being associated with chronic inflammation, it makes perfect sense that a healthy vegan diet could reduce the risk. With diverticular disease being described as a disease of fibre-deficiency,[168] a vegan diet could prevent it. A fibre-rich vegan diet would also, as we've already heard, influence the microbiome of the gut towards microbes that produce more short-chain fatty acids that are protective of the mucosal barrier and its role in immune function.[169] For these reasons, studies have shown that a high-fibre, mainly plant-based diet decreases the risk of diverticular disease[170] and a lower risk of admission to hospital or death from the condition.[171]

Constipation

Constipation describes the situation in which either stools are passed less frequently, or are hard and difficult to pass. It is a very common condition, with up to 20% of the adult population being affected by chronic constipation.[172] And although it sounds like quite a benign condition, the most recent 'Cost of Constipation' report stated that in 2018/19 almost 77,000 people were admitted to hospital due to constipation, and £168m was spent by the NHS on managing it.[173] These numbers are predicted to continue rising. If you have ever been constipated you will probably appreciate just how much it can affect your quality of life. It can be uncomfortable and inconvenient, but at its worst it can cause severe pain, and can sometimes result in tears in the back passage, and even rectal prolapse and bowel obstruction. Constipation has also been linked with urine retention, infections, and delerium in the elderly.

Whilst there are several causes of constipation, including medical conditions like hypothyroidism and some neurological disorders, and many medications like opioids and some antidepressants, lifestyle also plays a big part. Not moving around enough and not drinking sufficient water can both result in stubborn bowel movements, but not including enough plants in your diet will surely result in harder, less frequent stools. Of course, a healthy vegan diet is rich in fibre from all the of the plants consumed, so constipation and its complications will be far less likely when you are eating plant-based.

Irritable bowel syndrome

Irritable bowel syndrome, or IBS, is a very common condition which causes abdominal pains and alternating constipation and diarrhoea. People who suffer from IBS also report bloating and excess wind, and symptoms are sometimes triggered by eating, and improved with passing stools. The condition can get better or it can stay with you through life, but those who experience it often notice specific triggers, particularly in their diet, with dairy and gluten being common culprits. The cause of IBS isn't really known, although there does seem to be some association with previous infections with bacterial gastroenteritis, and stress and a family history of the condition also play a part. Once again, fibre comes into play, with it being common consensus that a low-fibre diet can lead to the development of IBS, but studies have shown that a high fibre intake can regulate the gut microbiome, producing those beneficial substances like butyrate, and reducing the risk of the condition.[174]

The mainstay of treatment for IBS is the Low FODMAP Diet. FODMAPs are types of carbohydrate that when ingested, can lead to IBS symptoms. They are **F**ermentable **O**ligo-saccharides, **D**i-saccharides, **M**ono-saccharides **A**nd **P**olyols. Most of the foods that contain these are fruits and vegetables, so in reducing the intake of these, the intake of fibre can also be reduced, worsening IBS in the long term. It is very possible, however, to reduce FODMAP intake, without becoming deficient in fibre. High fibre, low-FODMAP foods include gluten free oats, red lentils, chickpeas, kidney beans and rice. Many, many fruits and vegetables are also low-FODMAP, and you can find an extensive list of other such foods on a great fact sheet from the Plant Based Health Professionals UK.[175] Other pulses which are high in FODMAPs can also have their content reduced by soaking them, or using sprouting techniques. Interestingly, some dairy products also contain FODMAPS, like whole milk, Greek yoghurt, and processed cheeses, so some low FODMAP eating guides incorporate plant-based alternatives into their recommendations.[176]

A healthy plant-based diet which is low in FODMAPs could be a great way of managing IBS, as the increased fibre intake can re-regulate the microbiome, improve bowel health and reduce symptoms. But a sudden increase in fibre intake could worsen symptoms, temporarily, and increased intake should be done cautiously and carefully, perhaps with the help of a dietician.

Metabolic dysfunction-associated steatotic liver disease (MASLD)

I mentioned the mouthful that is metabolic dysfunction-associated steatotic liver disease earlier, in the context of its association with liver cancer. But let's talk about it a bit more here. Until recently, it was known as the equally tongue-twisting non-alcoholic fatty liver disease (NAFLD). This name makes a bit more sense to the non-expert, because it explains what is going on: the liver is fattier than it should be, but it isn't caused by alcohol intake (a very common culprit for liver disease). Its common name, which you might hear your GP mention, is just 'fatty liver', but this would also include alcohol as a potential cause. So what are the non-alcohol causes of a fatty liver? And why are we worried about a bit of fat in the liver?

The liver may be called upon to store excess fat because of obesity, raised triglyceride levels in the blood, and insulin resistance. In fact, some clinicians consider MASLD to be the liver-related manifestation of metabolic syndrome.[177] (To recap, metabolic syndrome is a cluster of conditions which occur together to increase the risk of type 2 diabetes, stroke and heart disease.) The reason why we're concerned about excess fat in the liver is because this storage, also known as steatosis, damages the cells of the liver, leading to liver fibrosis, cirrhosis, and a higher risk of hepatocellular carcinoma, or liver cancer. Thinking about the risk factors which contribute to this process, as for obesity, we know that vegans tend to have a lower BMI, so risk of MASLD would be expected to be lower, too. We've also read in the diabetes section all about how veganism reduces the risk of diabetes and improves insulin resistance, so that's another risk factor for MASLD reduced thanks to a vegan diet. Triglycerides are a type of dietary fat which are made by the liver from excess calories. In theory, if a vegan diet is lower in calorie density, and higher in fibre, it should also be lower risk for excess triglyceride production and storage, and therefore helpful for preventing MASLD. There isn't any firm evidence that a plant-based diet directly reduces blood triglyceride levels, however.

By tackling these risk factors, a healthy vegan diet really should lessen the likelihood of developing MASLD. One study did demonstrate that a healthy diet, rich in fruits, vegetables, nuts, antioxidants and minerals did seem to reduce this risk.[178] This intervention diet was described by the group in the study as being uncommon in the West, so it's probably not a surprise that whilst the prevalence of MASLD in Asia is somewhere between 5 and 18%, it is much higher in Western countries, being between 20 and 30%.[179]

Once again, plant-based diets are likely to be useful not just in risk reduction, but also in management of the condition once it is already established. The mainstay of MASLD treatment includes lifestyle changes that aim at weight loss,[180] and adherence to one particularly plant-rich diet, the EAT-Lancet reference diet, has been shown to be associated with both a reduced risk of developing MASLD, as well as its severity.[181]

EAT-Lancet Planetary Health Diet

The EAT-Lancet Commission involved scientists and experts from all over the planet, who were tasked with working out how we can feed a future population of 10 billion people a

healthy and sustainable diet. The global population is pre-
dicted to be at 10 billion by as soon as 2050, and when 733
million people faced hunger in 2023,[182] figuring out how to
ensure the number of those experiencing food insecurity is
reduced, or that famine is eliminated entirely, is a priority.
But this isn't as simple as it seems. The EAT-Lancet Commis-
sion also needed to consider how to do this within planetary
boundaries, and provide a healthful diet for all. So, they had
to consider things like the lifestyle related diseases that the
Western diet is causing, and the climate crisis to which ani-
mal agriculture is contributing.

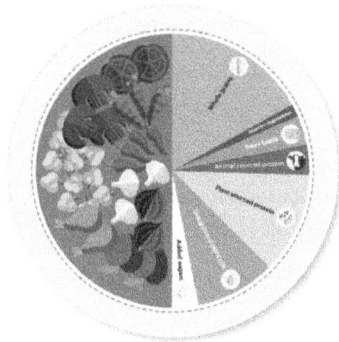

EAT-Lancet Planetary Health Diet

According to the commission, 'Transformation to healthy di-
ets by 2050 will require substantial dietary shifts. Global
consumption of fruits, vegetables, nuts and legumes will
have to double, and consumption of foods such as red meat
and sugar will have to be reduced by more than 50%. A
diet rich in plant-based foods and with fewer animal source
foods confers both improved health and environmental ben-
efits.'[183] To put into context what they recommend, the di-

agram above shows what a plate would look like when following their Planetary Health Diet.

Whilst dairy and animal sourced protein do have a small place on the Planetary Health Diet plate, they are optional, and were not deemed essential to human health after all of the evidence was reviewed. The reason why red meat was included, despite the commission acknowledging that the evidence shows that it is harmful to human health and the planet, is because there is little evidence of what happens in large groups of people who abstain entirely from consuming it. What the commission does recommend, however, is that if you are going to eat red meat, that you should do so in small quantities, at no more than 98g per week. Now, being a vegan, I had to research just how much red meat this is, as it doesn't sound like a lot at all. And it really isn't; the average steak is around 300g, so what is recommended here as a maximum intake is less than half a steak per week. Obviously I don't agree with this; when we take into account the experience of the victims of the meat industry, as well as the environmental and health impacts, meat has no place in the human diet.

Whether the diet will work in terms of protecting the environment and ending world hunger, only time will tell. But there are some studies which are beginning to demonstrate that the planetary diet may well have beneficial effects on our health. Studies have shown that the diet was associated with a reduced risk of cancer, and death from all causes,[184] as well as reducing the risk of diabetes, and that it could potentially be useful in managing T2DM.[185] The EAT-Lancet planetary health diet also seems to be beneficial in reducing the risk of depression and anxiety,[186] as well as reducing the *risk of cardiovascular disease by 14%, and ischaemic heart disease by 12%.[187]*

Further study into the possible associations between the EAT-Lancet diet and potential reductions in risk for various diseases are required, as the studies are still few in number, and there aren't large communities of people adopting this way of eating. But the commission predicted that if the diet was adopted globally, it could prevent 10.9 million deaths per year.

Bone Health

When I tell people I'm vegan, or I suggest to a patient that they could consider a trial of eliminating dairy, one question that comes up frequently is 'But won't that be bad for my bones?' It's no surprise, because dairy really has been pushed as the main source of calcium for a long time. I have discussed more about the problems and ethics of the dairy industry in the 'Vegan for the Animals' and 'Vegan for Social Justice' chapters, but here we'll address the question of dairy's role in bone health, and I'll reassure you that your bones don't need to suffer because you don't consume dairy.

The concerns with bone health are around bone density. Our bones are made from an inner matrix, onto which minerals are laid by specialised cells. Bones are continuously being broken down and remodelled by cells called osteoclasts and osteoblasts. Osteopenia and osteoporosis are conditions in which the bones are under-mineralised, causing weakness and a higher risk of fracture. The risk of osteoporosis increases significantly after menopause because the consequent lack of oestrogen means that the osteoclasts that break down and reabsorb bone tissue become more active in relation to the osteoblasts that build up bone tissue.

Osteopenia is the step before osteoporosis, and despite it sometimes being incidentally found on x-rays, to formally diagnose either condition, a bone density, or dexa, scan is needed. The minerals involved in strengthening bone matrix are primarily calcium and vitamin D, so diets deficient in these minerals could result in a lower bone density. Interestingly, having referred patients for many, many dexa scans because I'm concerned about bone density, I haven't once seen a tick box for 'vegan diet' as an indication for a dexa scan because it needn't be a risk factor for osteoporosis.

So what is the truth? What does the evidence show? And why were we all made to believe that we need to consume dairy? A nutrition scientist from Stanford University thinks it is because the dairy industry offered to pay for educational materials to schools for free, and wrongly included in that information that dairy is required in multiple servings per day.[188] But this was part of a wider propaganda project. A rise in dairy production and consumption really began to take off in the early twentieth century when US dairy farmers ramped up production in order to send high-nutrition milk products to Europe to support soldiers fighting in World War I.[189] The subsequent surplus of milk products instigated the widespread promotion of dairy as an essential health food, creating demand with policies like free milk for school children, and demand was met, resulting in a billion-dollar dairy industry in the US. I can't find a lot of information about how and why demand increased here in Europe, but American milk propaganda probably played a part; it wouldn't be the first or last time that British consumers have been influenced by American marketing and advertising campaigns. We also can't deny the fact that dairy seems to have a romantic image in the UK, with people nostalgically remembering deliveries of glass bottles of the white stuff by the milk-man, and images conjured of Jersey cows wandering freely around a beautiful, green, lush field.

The reality of modern dairy farming is far from this, though. Profit has certainly been a driver for association of milk and health in the UK; in the early twentieth century dairy farming was becoming Britain's most profitable agricultural sector,[190] and by 2025 the UK dairy industry was worth around £17.5 billion.[191]

It can't be denied that dairy does contain a whole host of nutrients, including protein, calcium and vitamin D, with most literature concentrating on the calcium aspect. But dairy isn't the only calcium-containing food. By a long stretch. I'll cover more details about calcium and which foods are rich in it in the Calcium section later in the book, but let's just say that somebody taking a varied vegan diet shouldn't need to worry too much about their calcium intake. And when we add to this understanding the fact that dairy contains harmful saturated fat and has been associated with many disease processes, as we've already read, relying on it as your source of calcium really isn't a good idea.

As for the evidence around bone health and plant-based diets, it is mixed and nuanced. One large study from the EPIC-Oxford group I have told you about before demonstrated that bone fractures were more frequent in vegans,[192] but they were also higher in pescatarians and vegetarians than in meat-eaters, suggesting that excluding dairy from the diet is not the issue. The researchers did comment that a lower BMI and reduced calcium intake in vegans could have contributed to the findings, but as we'll see later, calcium intake need not be lower in vegans, and a lower BMI, while it likely has an impact on bone health, reduces the risk of many other diseases. Another large UK study had similar findings, and concluded that the absolute difference in hip fracture meant there would only be an increase of around 3.2 more cases per 1000 people over 10 years, and that the reduced risk of cardiovascular disease which is associated with a vegetarian diet outweighed this risk.[193] The Adventist

Health Study-2 yielded results that back up the association with calcium intake, finding that while female vegans had a higher risk of hip fracture than non-vegetarians (the men in the study didn't), when calcium and vitamin D were supplemented, the risk went away.[194] One large US study of post-menopausal women, a group who are already at a higher risk of reduced bone density, found that a plant-based diet, whether healthy or unhealthy, was not associated with an increased risk of hip fractures.[195]

So, what appears to be important for bone health is that the intake of nutrients, such as calcium, protein, vitamins B12 and D is essential, but that being on a vegan diet doesn't mean that you have to be at higher risk of osteoporosis, because you can still ensure you are getting enough of these. I think we can even push to say that a healthy vegan diet, when supplemented with these nutrients, could even be beneficial for bone health, because soya has also been associated with a reduction in the risk of bone fracture by around one third in postmenopausal women,[196] probably owing to the effects of its isoflavones on oestrogen receptors, as we read about in the breast cancer section, which has beneficial effects on bone resorption and formation. Considering that vegans usually consume more soya products, this means we could reduce our risk of osteoporosis with a healthy, soy-rich vegan diet. Other important risk factors we must not forget when considering our bone health include minimising alcohol intake, avoiding smoking and taking regular weight-bearing exercise. Being mindful of all of this, and ensuring we are taking enough protein, calcium, and vitamins B12 and D, we can prevent detrimental effects on our bones from a plant-based diet, but also remember that we are reducing our overall risk of many other diseases.

Mental Health and Wellbeing

Although not always spoken about, mental health disorders are very common, with around 970 million people around the globe experiencing a mental health problem.[197] Whilst there is a lot of data around the impact of vegetarian and vegan diets on mental health, there is no clear association or evidence for either improved, or worsened mental health with any kind of diet. In fact, there is lots of evidence, but it is all rather conflicting.[198] What does seem to be the case, however, is that diet *quality* seems to affect mental wellbeing,[199] and once again, a 'good quality' diet is stated as being one which is rich in fruits, vegetables, nuts and wholegrains, and low in meat, amongst other harmful foods.[200] I'm never going to get bored of saying this, but fibre is likely key in this association. As we've learned in the obesity section, the diabetes section, the cardiovascular disease section, the cancer section, and the bowel section, fibre is an inflammation-reducing food, and some academics have postulated that inflammation may alter neurotransmitter concentrations, so by reducing inflammation we could improve the symptoms of depression.[201]

Other studies have suggested that the high polyphenol intake in a good plant-dominant diet could also be associated with a reduced prevalence of depression.[202] These healthful foods alter and enhance the microbiome, which could be beneficial for our mood considering that it has been demonstrated that patients with generalised anxiety disorder can have less microbial diversity in the gut, and fewer good bacteria that produce those really beneficial short-chain fatty acids.[203]

As well as the physical aspects that might connect mental health and veganism, I feel that the ethical considerations must play a part, too. If one considers veganism to be a philosophy, then you might feel a sense of belonging when you become vegan and 'join the gang'. It makes sense that a feeling of belonging can improve your emotional or mental wellbeing, but what's really interesting is that it can also have wondrous effects on your physical health, with a lack of belonging being associated with an increased risk of death.[204] It seems that keeping company can alter your gut microbiome,[205] but social exclusion can also negatively affect bowel flora.[206] Could inclusion into a group of people who teach compassion, kindness and love promote a microbiome that contributes to good health? Dr Gemma Newman, The Plant Power Doctor, certainly seems to think that a sense of belonging can improve your wellbeing. In her book *Get Well, Stay Well*, she shares her experiences of helping patients to feel this belonging by making sure they feel listened to and understood.[207] Which makes perfect sense, doesn't it? And I must say, that when I finally became vegan and found my tribe, I definitely felt more at ease, with myself and my decision. Conversely, finding that your moral compass has changed direction completely could leave you with a sense of loneliness if you aren't surrounded by others making the same transition, or who have already been through these changes. I'll be covering some tips for starting out on your vegan journey later, and I think finding other vegans to talk to and spend time with is an important part of staying well.

I also think there is a lot to say about the feeling of wellbeing that comes from a sense of purpose. There is evidence that backs this idea up, with several pieces of research showing a sense of purpose being protective from mental health disorders.[208] Whilst this purpose could come in many different forms, why shouldn't it be a cause that not only helps the plight of billions of animals around the world, but could also serve to slow down or halt the climate crisis. Personally, I think it would hard to find another motivation that feels quite so enormous, and full of hope.

Changing your behaviours so that your morals and actions become aligned could also have a positive effect on your wellbeing. Cognitive dissonance is a way of describing the discomfort an individual can feel when their actions and beliefs are incongruent; wouldn't this be a perfect way to describe many meat eaters? Most people would call themselves animal lovers. But still they purchase and consume products that have come from the enslavement, slaughter and exploitation of non-human animals. Cognitive dissonance can feel like anxiety, or distress, and the cause may not be immediately recognised by the person experiencing it. But I think the anger and aggression that vegans face from others when talking about why we don't eat animals could be cognitive dissonance rearing its head.

Even if you don't necessarily have these feelings of dissonance, merely realigning your moral compass and living by a set of principles such as veganism, could improve your sense of wellbeing. Whilst morality is thought to be associated with happiness,[209] having a clear moral identity is also thought to be essential for feeling that sense of purpose we were discussing earlier,[210] and thus improving your overall wellbeing.

Menopause

Whilst the menopause isn't a chronic disease, it is often a significant stretch of time in the lives of many people where there can be difficult symptoms, and so I include it here. Not all are troubled by the potential symptoms of peri- and menopause, but for those who are, they can be potentially life-changing, often requiring medications like HRT (hormone replacement therapy), but there are lifestyle measures that can improve the experience of menopause, and there is some evidence that a plant-based diet can help.

Menopause describes the time in a person's life when levels of oe-strogen decline to the point that their periods stop, and they are no longer fertile. The lead up to this, which can last for several years, is called *perimenopause*, and some of the symptoms that occur with and after menopause can occur during this time, too. Once somebody has gone through menopause, they are called post-menopausal, and they won't have had a period for at least one year. Although this is a normal life stage, it is important to remember that some people can experience this much earlier than the average age range of 45 to 55 years old, and it can also result from surgery or some cancer treatments, rather than just occurring naturally. Oestro-gen is the reproductive hormone which is responsible for typically female sexual characteristics, so it is women and people who are born with ovaries that experience this stage of life.

The symptoms of menopause include amenorrhoea (no peri-ods), but it's also not that unusual for people to experience menor-rhagia (heavy periods) or irregular bleeding in the perimenopause. Vasomotor symptoms – hot flushes and night sweats – occur in around 80% of people experiencing menopause,[211] and other symp-toms include mood changes, irritability, brain fog, vaginal dryness, insomnia, reduced libido and aches and pains.

It has been reported that vegans experience fewer of the troubling vasomotor symptoms,[212] and some studies have even demonstrated that adopting a vegan diet can reduce symptoms like hot flushes con-siderably in those already experiencing them.[213] This can be due to a higher intake of soya products. Soya is rich in isoflavones, which we have already seen are a form of phytoestrogen, and a typical serv-ing of soya food can contain around 25mg of isoflavones.[214] It seems to be these isoflavones which are beneficial in treating menopausal symptoms,[215] but that they must contain one particular isoflavone called genistein.[216] Soya isn't just beneficial for the vasomotor symptoms of menopause, but along with all of its many health benefits, it also seems to be protective against bone fractures in postmenopausal women,[195] and as discussed in the bone health section, the risk of osteoporosis increases greatly after menopause.

Whilst it is clear that plant-based foods can help with symptoms of menopause, modern HRT medications are now very safe, and the small increase in risk of certain adverse effects like breast cancer are very often outweighed by the big increase in quality of life experienced by those who taken them. It is worth having a conversation with your GP about starting HRT if you are menopausal and keen to try it, but the evidence shows that a fibre- and soya-rich vegan diet could be very beneficial alongside any treatment you decide to have. It could also be worth considering that your risk of some of the cancers that are associated with HRT might already be lower because of your healthy vegan diet, but this should be discussed with your clinician.

Chronic Kidney Disease

Chronic kidney disease (CKD) describes a reduced kidney function, and can happen for many reasons. The kidneys work to filter our blood, and we measure how well they are doing this with two tests: a blood test called eGFR, or estimated glomerular filtration rate, and urine ACR (albumin:creatinine ratio). The glomeruli are little collections of blood vessels in the kidneys which filter the blood plasma through to the tubes of the kidney where it can be excreted or reabsorbed; by measuring how well they are doing this, we can see how efficiently the kidneys are working. Creatinine is a waste product in our blood, so as the filtration rate goes down, or the kidney's efficiency reduces, the creatinine level rises.

Risk factors for developing CKD include obesity, hypertension, diabetes and cardiovascular disease, so before we even begin to delve into how plant-based eating could be beneficial specifically for kidney health, we can see that by its protective properties in relation to these conditions, a vegan diet could be useful in the primary prevention of CKD. And several studies seem to demonstrate that people who follow a vegan diet do seem to have a lower incidence of CKD compared with omnivores,[217,218] even in those who already had a higher risk of CKD,[219] and it can reduce the decline in kidney function that can occur over time.

But apart from the cardiovascular and metabolic benefits of a vegan diet that can reduce the risk of developing CKD, it seems that plant-based diets can have other positive effects which could make them useful in those who already have CKD; in other words, for secondary prevention. It has been understood for a long time that a high protein intake could be harmful to damaged kidneys because it puts pressure on a renal system which is already strained. Whilst vegan diets are sometimes (wrongly) criticised for always being lower in protein content, this is one scenario in which a lower protein intake could be useful, and plant-based diets have been described as safe and easily allowing for an intentional reduction in protein intake when compared with omnivorous diets.[220]

Further benefits are gained from — you guessed it — the high fibre content of a healthy vegan diet. It has been described how a high-fibre diet can improve the damage done to the gut microbiome associated with CKD, and increase the production of polyunsaturated fatty acids like butyrate, providing the gut microbes with energy so that amino acids reaching the colon can be incorporated into bacterial proteins and excreted. These amino acids, the building blocks of proteins, would otherwise be absorbed into the bloodstream, but if they were excreted in stools, they could bypass the kidneys and avoid putting further pressure on them.[221] The higher fibre intake of a plant-based diet can also improve gut motility. Again, this can reduce the amount of time amino acids are sitting around in the colon being fermented, but also any resultant toxins which could be harmful to the kidneys won't be sitting around in the colon long enough to be absorbed. Interestingly, chronic constipation has been demonstrated to be a risk factor for both the development and progression of CKD.[222] The low-inflammatory nature of a healthy vegan diet once again makes an appearance, as low grade inflammation and oxidative stress are commonly found in CKD,[223] but it's also the acidic nature of a Western diet rich in animal proteins and low in fruits and vegetables, that can hasten a complication of CKD called metabolic acidosis.[224] This could mean that a more alkali, vegan diet could be more kidney-healthy by reducing the acid-load.

It is for all of these reasons that a diet richer in plant proteins rather than animal-derived proteins has been associated with a lower mortality in those with CKD,[225] and it seems that previous concerns about the risk of a high potassium intake from fruits and vegetables, which would be harmful to a kidney no longer equipped to deal with it, don't seem to be a real issue, because plant-based diets don't seem to induce hyperkalaemia in CKD patients.[226,227] The increased sodium content of processed vegan foods could be problematic, however,[228] but in a whole-food plant-based diet, or at least a healthy vegan one, this really shouldn't be an issue.

Dementia

Dementia is an umbrella term for several conditions which cause memory loss, cognitive difficulties, behaviour changes, and reduced functioning. This can affect daily activities and even simple things like eating and dressing. These conditions are progressive and irreversible, and usually related to old age, although they can also occur in much younger people. The main cause of dementia is Alzheimer's disease, which accounts for 50–75% of dementia cases,[229] but other causes include vascular, Lewy body, and frontotemporal dementias. Both Alzheimer's and vascular dementia share many of the lifestyle-related risk factors that keep cropping up in this chapter: hypertension, high cholesterol, cardiovascular disease and obesity.

For this reason, it comes as no surprise that some of the healthier eating patterns have been associated with brain health and a reduced risk of dementia.[230] Diets which have been shown to be beneficial, such as the Mediterranean, DASH (Dietary Approaches to Stop Hypertension), and MIND (Mediterranean-DASH Intervention for Neurodegenerative Delay), all have the common properties of being low in saturated fats and sugar, high in fruits, vegetables, whole grains and nuts, and low in red and processed meat. As with other diseases we've already read about in this chapter, eliminating saturated fats and animal proteins confers a benefit to brain health. It reduces our exposure to inflammation and other harmful substances like TMAO (trimethylamine N-oxide), a metabolite of meat, and is thought to be implicated specifically in the disease process of Alzheimer's.[231]

But, once again, it's also the addition of healthy substances from fruits and vegetables that seem to help in *reducing* the risk of dementias.[232] And again, it seems to be the phytochemicals that confer an antioxidant benefit, because oxidative stress has been shown to be implicated in the development of dementia, which antioxidants could counteract.[233] Furthermore, healthy plant foods have effects on the gut microbiome which could influence the risk of developing Alzheimer's disease.[234]

Whilst there is very little evidence informing us about the effects of a purely plant-based or vegan diet on either the risk of developing dementia, or in slowing it down in those who are already diagnosed, some studies have shown an association between a largely plant-based diet and a lower risk in certain populations.[235,236] But these diets have often contained small amounts of either red meat or fish. I think for this reason, a small amount of fish is still advocated for by some, in terms of neurological health, but when we can supplement fish-specific nutrients like omega-3, the planetary effects of fishing along with the cruelty it involves need to be considered before including fish in your diet.

What's clear, though, is that more research needs to be done into exploring what effects a WFPB diet could have on the risk of dementia. It also needs to be said that, along with omega-3, we need to make sure that we supplement our vegan diet with vitamin B12, because deficiency of this micronutrient specifically is known to have deleterious effects on the central nervous system, potentially causing dementia-type symptoms, and as you will read later, B12 is impossible to obtain in unfortified vegan foods.

Skin

Acne

Acne is an inflammatory skin condition in which there is excessive production of sebum, causing lesions like comedones (blackheads) and inflammatory pustules. These result in pain, scarring, and embarrassment. It is a condition which affects primarily teenagers who are going through significant hormonal changes, but it can occur through to later stages of life in some people. There are various treatments including topical creams, oral antibiotics, and even the contraceptive pill, and when these fail, GPs can refer patients with acne to a dermatologist, who might start a medication called Roaccutane.

This is reserved for the severest of cases, because it can have some serious side effects, and needs to be taken with a lot of caution.

Whilst many clinicians will inform their patients that there is no proven link between acne and the diet, just anecdotally I can say that in my practice many patients notice that their skin improves when they cut dairy out of their diet. And although there aren't any big studies exploring the association, there is some evidence in the data that there could, indeed, be a link. Various studies have shown an association between milk consumption and an increased prevalence of acne,[237-239] and there are probably several reasons for this. One is down to the hormonal impacts of milk consumption. Acne is driven by hormones including androgens and IGF-1. Androgens are hormones that are responsible for primarily male sexual characteristics, and IGF-1 might sound familiar because we covered it in the cancer section, in the context of dairy potentially being associated with prostate malignancies. Levels of both IGF-1 and insulin are thought to be higher in those who consume dairy,[240] and increased insulin levels can drive hyperandrogenism, also potentially being mechanistic in the acne disease process. Whey and casein, the protein components of milk, have also been associated with increased levels of IGF-1 and insulin,[241] possibly also contributing to this link between acne and dairy.

But it isn't just the dairy in our diets that is likely to be increasing the risk of acne. Globally, as diets become more westernised, acne prevalence increases, and this seems to be in part due to the high glycaemic index of foods consumed in the West.[242] Just to recap, glycaemic index (GI) is the measure of a food's ability to alter your blood sugar, with those that have a low GI having the least impact, and high GI foods causing blood sugars to rise rapidly and higher. Increased risk is likely due to a combination of the effects of an increased dairy intake and the generally higher glycaemic index of an omnivorous diet, and acne patients have been shown to be twice as likely to have a non-vegan diet.[243] So, it's not too surprising that a healthy vegan one could be recommended as being beneficial for preventing and reducing acne lesions.[244] We should also bear in mind the association between obesity and acne; people with obesity tend to have higher levels of androgen, insulin and IGF-1,[245] meaning that the positive effects of a vegan diet on BMI could also be beneficial from this point of view.

Once again, the benefits of a vegan diet on skin health aren't just due to the abstinence from harmful animal-derived foods, but we can probably attribute some of the effects to the low-inflammatory nature of plant-based eating. As we keep discovering, a diet that cuts out red meat, dairy, highly processed foods and refined sugar has fewer inflammatory effects on the body, but the fibre-rich nature of it will also be influential on the gut microbiome in such a way that has also been thought to affect the skin. Evidence suggests that the gut microbiome can play an important part in the development of acne, and that plant-based foods could be used as a way of managing it.[246] As well as the wonderful organic chemicals like polyphenols found in lots of plant foods, it also seems that soya, specifically, could be really useful in those suffering from acne[247] and one study demonstrated that when 160mg of soya bean isoflavones was given as a medication to patients with acne for 12 weeks, there was a significant reduction in the number of acne lesions.[248] The positive effects of soya on acne symptoms is likely due to the way that it affects the hormone receptors in the human body.

Eczema

Eczema is another inflammatory skin condition and it presents as red, itchy scaly lesions, usually in the creases of skin behind the knees and near the elbows, but you can get these anywhere. It's really common in children, but can occur at any age, and there are lots of causes but it is often due to an allergic reaction to either something the skin has come into contact with, or with something that's been eaten.

There isn't a huge amount of evidence of the effects of diet, including a vegan one, on eczema, but some studies do show a benefit. It is worth considering that, as eczema is an inflammatory condition which can be associated with allergies, a healthy plant-based diet could be useful because it can be rich in flavanoids – metabolites of polyphenols – which are antioxidant *and* can have anti-allergic properties.[249] The influence of these on the gut microbiome could also have further anti-inflammatory effects as there is evidence that microbiome health, which we know is associated with what we eat, can impact on conditions like eczema.[250]

Children who are diagnosed with CMPA (cow's milk protein allergy) can also experience atopic eczema as part of their collection of symptoms. If you suspect this in your child, then make an appointment to discuss it with your doctor, because more tests might be needed, and other causes will need to be considered by your GP. Obviously, a vegan diet would remove this trigger, or make it so that it was never a problem in the first place, but it is important to note that soya allergy is often also found in those allergic to cow's milk, so caution may need to be taken with children who switch to a plant-based diet who were previously diagnosed with CMPA.

Psoriasis

Psoriasis is another inflammatory skin condition, which, like eczema, results in red scaly patches, but psoriasis isn't usually quite as itchy as eczema. It's also often distributed differently, and plaques are very often seen on the outer aspects of the elbows, on the kneecaps, or behind the ears and in the posterior hair line. Where eczema is often a reaction to something the person has come into contact with, psoriasis is autoimmune, which I'll explain further on in this chapter.

Whilst there isn't very much research showing associations between plant-based eating and psoriasis, it is worth considering the underlying causes of psoriasis. We know that it is an inflammatory condition, with links to autoimmune disease. We have read, time and time again, that a healthy vegan diet is an anti-inflammatory one. So even without much evidence, it would be fair to assume that a plant-based diet could help with managing the symptoms of psoriasis, due to the low-inflammatory properties of this way of eating. It is also important to recognise that psoriasis is known to be associated with obesity, cardiovascular disease and type 2 diabetes.[251] With a sound evidence base that a healthy vegan diet can help to reduce the risk of these conditions, we could at least prevent some of the potential risk factors for psoriasis, or reduce their impact in those who are more likely to suffer from them. Then there is also the fact that dairy, sugar, meat and eggs have been named as triggers for psoriasis by those with the condition.[252] So perhaps, despite a lack of reliable studies up to now, there is enough evidence surrounding the associated conditions and risk factors that it could be worth considering a healthy vegan diet to reduce the impact of psoriasis on your health.

Hidradenitis suppurativa

Hidradenitis suppurativa (HS) is a debilitating skin condition which causes pus-filled lesions and abscesses in the skin, resulting in infections, pain and scarring. The lesions occur wherever there is a higher number of sweat glands, so under the arms, the groins and lower abdomen are most frequently affected. Acute lesions usually need to be managed with antibiotics to treat the infection, but surgery is often required to deal with the lesions, too, as well as the complications they can cause.

As with many of the conditions we've discussed already, there is potential for a vegan diet to help prevent flare-ups because of the inflammatory nature of HS, meaning it could gain benefit from an anti-inflammatory pattern of eating. As it is also associated with hypertension, obesity, type 2 diabetes and raised lipids, amongst other conditions,[253] there is potential for a healthy vegan diet, which is known to be beneficial in reducing the risk of these conditions, to lower the risk of developing HS, or to reduce its negative effects.

The one condition that HS seems to be most closely associated with is obesity. As we've already read, obesity leads to insulin resistance and increased insulin levels. Alongside higher levels of IGF-1, and a rise in androgens, insulin stimulates androgen receptors that increase keratin production in the skin, blocking hair follicles and causing the inflammation that can result in acne and HS.[254] For this reason, managing obesity, which can be a contributor to the development and worsening of HS, could help to reduce the symptoms. And it isn't just managing obesity as a risk factor that could make vegan eating beneficial to those with HS; removing dairy from the diet could specifically have positive effects, as it has been linked to a worsening of HS symptoms.[255] It also seems that a healthy dairy-free and low GI diet could improve symptoms and prevent it from worsening, with one small study showing an improvement when dairy was eliminated.[256] It is likely that the direct effect of IGF-1 from the milk itself, along with other elements such as casein and whey, impact the glands and hair follicles resulting in HS lesions.[257]

Once again, those little bugs in our gut probably have an effect too. Evidence shows that HS can result when the gut microbiome goes out of balance.[258] As we know, the more plants and fibre that we eat, the better the health of our microbiome, so this is another way in which eating vegan could reduce the effects and symptoms of HS. Some deficiencies have been linked with HS, primarily zinc and vitamin D,[259] and while we do know that vitamin D deficiency is a risk with plant-based eating, as we will discuss in the 'Staying Well' chapter, this is easily prevented and treated with supplementation. Interestingly, supplementation of not just vitamin D and zinc have been associated with an improvement in symptoms of HS, but taking more omega-3 fatty acids could also be beneficial.[260] As you will read later, omega-3 ought to be taken into account when planning our vegan meals and nutrient intake.

Autoimmune Diseases

Rheumatoid arthritis

Rheumatoid arthritis is an inflammatory arthritis, caused by autoimmune disease. This means that there is a fault in the immune system, causing it to wrongly target the body's own tissues. In the case of rheumatoid arthritis this results in pain, swelling and destruction of the soft tissues around the joints. It usually starts in the small joints of the hands and feet, but can go on to affect bigger joints and other organs including the heart, lungs and eyes. You may have noticed somebody with hands that have been damaged by rheumatoid arthritis, as they can end up with quite marked deformities with the fingers pointing outwards. As well as the pain associated with flare-ups, the other reason for treating rheumatoid arthritis adequately and as early as possible, is to prevent these deformities which can result in disability. But does a plant-based diet play a part in managing or preventing the condition?

The anti-inflammatory nature of a healthy vegan diet should have positive effects on the symptoms of a condition like rheumatoid arthritis, especially when we consider that risk factors for developing the disease probably include changes in the microbiome and a Western diet.[261] And, indeed, some studies do show that a vegan diet, along with other anti-inflammatory eating patterns like vegetarian and the Mediterranean diets, can improve symptoms like pain.[262] The elimination of animal-derived foods certainly could be part of the solution, as it has been shown that the high consumption of these foods is associated with the development of rheumatoid arthritis.[263,264]

A plant-based diet could also benefit those at risk of or already diagnosed with rheumatoid arthritis because of its positive effects on BMI. We already know about the lower risk of obesity with a vegan diet, and that there is an association between high BMI and the risk of developing rheumatoid arthritis.[265] This is, in part, because excess fat releases inflammatory substances called adipokines which lead to tissue inflammation.[266] However, it isn't just the association with obesity for which removing harmful animal products is beneficial, but also the impact of cholesterol on the development of rheumatoid arthritis. There is some evidence from one large study that a raised cholesterol, which we know is found only in animal-derived foods, could lead to rheumatoid arthritis in women, although the same result wasn't found in men.[267]

I'm sure that by now you have noticed that I keep coming back to the same themes: a vegan diet reduces or eliminates harmful substances and ingredients, but also adds beneficial ones. And it is because of this that I can go on to tell you that a healthy plant-based diet could offer further perks for somebody with rheumatoid arthritis because of the inclusion of wonderful substances like polyphenols, which have been shown to help reduce inflammation in conditions like theirs.[268] In addition, the increased fibre intake in a vegan diet can increase the production of anti-inflammatory SCFAs and reduce harmful substances, like cytokines, through its effect on the microbiome.[269] It is for this reason that a vegan diet rich in fruits, vegetables, and without animal products has been shown to have potential benefit for reducing the risk of autoimmune conditions like rheumatoid arthritis.[270]

I should issue a word of caution, however. Of the few deficiencies that are a bigger risk for vegans, one of them is vitamin D. There is some evidence that a lack of vitamin D could lead to the development of rheumatoid arthritis.[271] As such, amongst many other reasons, it's important that those following the vegan lifestyle should supplement with a vegan vitamin D product. I'll go into this in more detail in the 'Staying Well' chapter. It's also worth mentioning here, although it isn't specific to veganism because many people, including omnivores, simply aren't getting enough, but omega-3 is also really important. Again, I'll discuss what this is in much more detail in the next section of the book, but omega-3s are a type of fatty acid which are found most frequently in fish, so as vegans, we can run the risk of not consuming enough. Taking higher quantities of omega-3 fatty acids has been shown to reduce the production of inflammatory substances like cytokines, and are therefore useful in the management of rheumatoid arthritis.[272] As we will read about later, as vegans we really need to consider our intake of omega-3 fatty acids, so supplementing with an algae-derived source can be really useful.

One final point is that people with rheumatoid arthritis are twice as likely to suffer from cardiac disease,[273] so reducing your risk with lifestyle measures such as a healthy vegan diet could help to mitigate some of this risk, or least make sure you are not adding to it with harmful, heart-disease associated, animal-derived foods.

Psoriatic arthritis

Psoriatic arthritis is another autoimmune joint disease, which can present similarly to rheumatoid arthritis, as described above. It is similar in the sense that there can be pain, stiffness and swelling. It can occur with or without psoriasis, the skin disease I previously told you about, which causes thickened, scaly plaques. Like rheumatoid arthritis, it can also cause destruction of the joints, and should be caught early to prevent or reduce the disability that can ensue.

There is very little evidence for the impact of a vegan diet on psoriatic arthritis. That said, being an inflammatory condition, and given everything that we've already learned about how a healthy vegan diet can benefit those with or at risk of inflammatory conditions, it would make sense that eating plant-based could help. One case report has been published, however, and it just so happens to be about a fellow member of Plant-Based Health Professionals: Kate Dunbar was diagnosed with psoriatic arthritis, and was treated with a strong medication, called methotrexate[274]. She reports that 14 years after diagnosis, she decided to start a WFPB diet. Less than a year later she was able to stop her medication completely, remaining off it ever since, with good symptom control.

Whilst there have been no studies investigating whether there is a role for plant-based diets in treating and preventing psoriatic arthritis, it comes as no surprise that there is data to show that a Mediterranean diet can reduce inflammation and improve disease activity.[275-277] This is partly due to its association with obesity, which is a known risk factor for the development of psoriatic arthritis,[278] but also because of its anti-inflammatory properties. For this reason, I don't think that it would be a huge leap to suggest that a plant-based diet could have similar effects. But at the very least, it could help with managing BMI and therefore reducing the risk of developing the condition, and with mitigating the increased risk of cardiovascular disease that, much like rheumatoid arthritis, often comes with the condition.

Thyroid disease

The thyroid gland is a little mass of tissue that sits low down on the front of the throat. It produces thyroid hormone, and is stimulated to do this by a hormone released from the pituitary gland in the brain, called thyroid stimulating hormone (TSH). Thyroid hormone works to increase the rate at which your cells work, and is also implicated in normal growth and mental development. There are many different types of thyroid disease, some causing overactivity of the gland, or hyperthyroidism, and others causing it to slow down and become sluggish, known as hypothyroidism. Both hyperthyroidism and hypothyroidism have multiple causes, but both can be caused by autoimmune disease. This is what I will discuss here.

Hypothyroidism

The most common cause of an underactive thyroid is autoimmune thyroiditis, or Hashimoto's disease, which sees the immune system depositing immune cells into the tissue of the thyroid gland. Whilst obesity has been identified as a cause of this condition, it is actually a bidirectional relationship: obesity impacts thyroid health, again partly due to the pro-inflammatory nature of a raised BMI,[279] but a reduced thyroid function will almost certainly cause weight gain. Therefore, it makes sense that a plant-based diet could reduce the risk of Hashimoto's disease, because of its association with a lower BMI, but also because of the lower levels of inflammatory markers seen in vegans. Although one study showed a weak association between a vegan diet and some protection against hypothyroidism,[280] there is currently very little data on the effects of plant-based eating on the disease. It is mentioned here because of the potential effects of a vegan diet, in view of the fact that it is an autoimmune condition, therefore has inflammatory associations, and could benefit from a low-inflammatory diet such as the vegan one.

It is also important to mention that hypothyroidism, in particular congenital hypothyroidism, is associated with iodine deficiency. Whilst autoimmune disease is the most common cause of hypothyroidism in the West, in developing countries the main cause is iodine deficiency due to endemically low soil iodine levels, meaning that crops grown in those places are also low in the mineral. Iodine is vital for thyroid hormone production, but I'll explain more about this later. Iodine, as you will find out, is one of the micronutrients that I recommend that vegans supplement alongside our diet. This could help to prevent deficiency-related hypothyroidism and congenital hypothyroidism seen in babies.

Hyperthyroidism

Whilst autoimmune disease can cause an underactive thyroid, it is also often responsible for overactivity, with Grave's disease being the most common cause of hyperthyroidism. Again, the immune system attacks the tissues of the thyroid gland, but this time they cause stimulation and over-production of thyroid hormone. There is a dearth of evidence about the effects of a plant-based diet on preventing and managing hyperthyroidism, but one very large study did show a lower prevalence of hyperthyroidism in those who didn't consume animal-derived foods, with vegans having 52% lower odds of a hyperthyroidism diagnosis compared with those who ate animal products.[281] This is, again, likely due to the reduction in inflammation associated with vegan eating. Theoretically, excess iodine intake could cause hyperthyroidism but this is extremely rare.

Osteoarthritis

Osteoarthritis, whilst also being a disease of the joints, is different from rheumatoid arthritis and psoriatic arthritis, in that it isn't caused by autoimmunity, and is driven by wear and tear of the articular surfaces of the joint. Osteoarthritis has always been thought of as a degenerative joint condition rather than an inflammatory process, but read on to find out how this has changed in recent times.

Osteoarthritis occurs when the nice, healthy cartilage layer protecting the joint-facing surface of a bone becomes thin and worn, causing pain within the joint. Flare-ups can cause localised inflammation around the affected joint, with swelling, warmth and tenderness or pain on moving the joint. It is a very common condition with around 10 million people in the UK being affected,[282] and it usually affects older adults, although the onset can be earlier in some. The most common risks factors are age, sex, previous injuries to the joint, obesity, and a family history.

Once again, we see obesity being implicated in yet another disease process, potentially offering another way in which a plant-based diet could help. Through weight reduction, or reducing the risk of obesity in the first place, you could lessen the impact on the affected joints, as it's the weight-bearing joints, like the hips and knees, that are often affected first. For example, a greater body weight puts more pressure on the knee joints when mobilising, and so this contributes to the disease process of joint degeneration in osteoarthritis. It's simple mechanics, really. The space between the bones of the knee, which should be filled with synovial fluid that keeps the joint lubricated and moving smoothly, reduces due to the pressure of extra weight on top of it, pushing the bones together, and eventually the cartilage surfaces rub together for so long that they wear out.

This process has been accepted for a long time as the primary mechanism in the development of osteoarthritis. But what about the joints that aren't weight bearing? What about those at the ends of the fingers, which are commonly affected by osteoarthritis? Well, it is now understood that the low-grade systemic inflammation related to obesity, which sees the secretion of pro-inflammatory adipokines and cytokines, contributes to the degeneration seen in joints affected by osteoarthritis.[283,284] It is for this reason that anti-inflammatory diets such as a healthy vegan diet could positively impact the disease process of osteoarthritis, in addition to its influence over BMI and obesity. And, in fact, it has been demonstrated that the Mediterranean diet, rich in polyphenols, can prevent inflammation and cartilage destruction, preventing osteoarthritis-related disease activity in the joint,[285] and even improve quality of life in those who have it.[286]

It is also worth noting the fact that metabolic conditions like raised cholesterol, high blood pressure and insulin resistance have been associated with an increased risk of developing osteoarthritis, with the prevalence of metabolic syndrome in those with osteoarthritis being found to be around 59%, compared with just 23% in the general population.[287] So, if we can see evidence that the Mediterranean diet can help with osteoarthritis, is there a role for a healthy vegan diet? One small study did show that a WFPB diet resulted in significant reduction in pain very soon after starting to eat plant-based,[288] but unfortunately we have very little other evidence, because no studies have been carried out. But when we have seen that reduction in weight and inflammation could help, and there is suggestion that meat consumption is associated with degenerative joint disease,[289] it would make sense that osteoarthritis could be yet another chronic condition that could benefit from a healthy vegan lifestyle. Increased fibre intake once again plays its part, with there being evidence that it could lead to a reduction in the impact of symptoms in osteoarthritis.[290]

Migraine

Migraine is a very common condition which causes headaches that are usually associated with nausea, vomiting and photophobia. It often comes with 'aura' which are neurological symptoms, like visual disturbance or a change in sensation or weakness in a limb. The frequency and severity of migraine varies wildly, with some people having a short episode, lasting just an hour or two, whereas others can end up in bed for several days with their migraines. For some, the symptoms of migraine can be very disabling, even causing stroke-like symptoms.

Many people with migraine will be able to tell you about triggers for their episodes, which are often food and drink related. Common triggers are chocolate, alcohol and caffeine, but with dairy also being reported by some as a trigger,[291] perhaps a healthy vegan diet could play a role in preventing episodes, or reducing symptoms? There certainly is some evidence that a healthy diet could reduce the frequency of attacks, with a typical Western diet being associated with a higher frequency.[292] And healthy diets, including plant-based, DASH, and Mediterranean, seem to be associated with reduced symptoms of migraine related headaches,[293] but the evidence for a purely plant-based diet in managing migraines does remain limited. One small study showed a reduction in migraine related pain with a plant-based diet,[294] and they suggested that possible mechanisms include the removal of triggers like dairy, the low-inflammatory nature of a vegan diet, and the weight reduction that often comes with plant-based eating. An association has also been made between obesity and migraine,[295] meaning that a healthy vegan diet could also be of benefit because of its effects on metabolic syndrome and its cardiovascular consequences.[296] As you may recall, metabolic syndrome includes the conditions of hypertension, raised cholesterol, and type 2 diabetes, on all of which plant-based diets can have a positive effect.

There may be other factors at play, too. One way in which healthy vegan eating could help is that it is a diet often lower in sodium, which can trigger migraines. Also many vegetables contain chemicals which can reduce the effects of calcitonin gene-related peptide (CGRP), a protein thought to be implicated in the mechanism of migraines by causing inflammation in the nervous system.[292] Low-fat diets are also thought to reduce headache frequency, intensity and duration in those with migraines,[297] and, seeing as magnesium deficiency has been implicated in the mechanism of migraine onset,[298] the potentially higher intake of magnesium, which is abundant in many whole-foods, could help. Finally, the hormonal effects of a vegan diet, as discussed earlier in the chapter, could have some effect on migraine, because for some, fluctuations in oestrogen can influence migraine symptoms.[299]

How animals set me on a path to healing
Dr Leila Dehghan-Zaklaki
www.plantedacademy.com

For as long as I can remember, migraines not only controlled my life but defined me as a person. They were my dark secret, something I didn't want others to know because I feared it would make me seem weak or undesirable – as a friend, colleague, or person. Eventually, the migraines became so debilitating that I had to leave my career as a paediatrician – a job I truly loved. After losing the security and status my profession gave me, my confidence hit rock bottom.

During this time, I got involved in dog rescue work. Through this work, I learned the truth about animal agriculture: the systemic exploitation and suffering inflicted on animals for human consumption and entertainment. Once I understood the suffering behind my food choices, I couldn't ignore it and went vegan overnight. But unlike some lucky vegans, cutting out dairy didn't bring relief for my migraines. Over time, my migraines only got worse, and eventually, they became chronic. I was suffering up to 18 days a month, with 10 of those days spent bedridden in excruciating pain.

A vegan diet might not have initially improved my health, but it set me on the path to healing. At the time, I was working as a personal trainer, and clients constantly asked me where I got my protein as a vegan. To answer their questions, I began researching nutrition, and that's when I discovered the whole-food, plant-based (WFPB) diet. In desperation, I decided to try it, shifting from junk food to nutrient-dense, unprocessed plant foods. Within just five days, my migraines disappeared – it felt miraculous. But I was also frustrated: why hadn't I been taught this in medical school? How could something so powerful and accessible not be part of mainstream medicine?

This transformation didn't just restore my health; it completely redefined the course of my life. Determined to understand the science behind my experience, I pursued a master's degree in nutrition. What I learned amazed me: a plant-based diet not only supports good health but also helps prevent chronic disease. At the same time, it eliminates the need for animal cruelty by removing animals from the food system altogether.

Today, I work as an educator because I believe knowledge is the most powerful tool for change. I create courses and resources to help others understand the transformative potential of a whole-food, plant-based lifestyle. What once felt like the worst thing that could happen – losing my career to migraines – turned out to be a blessing in disguise. My own health challenges led me to discover the power of plant-based eating, which I now promote as a way to help people as well as animals.

What's more, the ripple effects of this lifestyle go far beyond individual benefits. A plant-based diet advances health equity, food justice, and environmental sustainability. While my migraines no longer define me, they have undoubtedly shaped me, and I'm grateful for where they've led me today.

Polycystic Ovarian Syndrome

Polycystic ovarian syndrome (PCOS), is a condition that describes ovaries with many cysts on them, alongside either reduced or no periods (oligomenorrhoea/amenorrhoea), and/or signs of hyperandrogenism, like hirsutism (increased hair growth on the body or face), acne, hair loss, or blood tests showing increased levels of androgens. It is often diagnosed after a patient complains of their periods either stopping or becoming infrequent, and the other symptoms, if present, are noted, but often not the primary concern. PCOS is a worry for several reasons: for the patient who is often worried about their fertility, and for both the patient and the clinician, because it is usually associated with metabolic syndrome, putting them at increased risk of conditions like heart disease and type 2 diabetes.

PCOS is very often associated with obesity, although we're not entirely sure of the full mechanism. We do know, however, that continued obesity drives the process, and worsening of the symptoms because of how it increases androgen levels. Therefore the Recommendations from the International Evidence-based Guideline for the Assessment and Management of PCOS advises weight management as one the main treatment strategies.[300]

The other way in which weight loss helps in the management of PCOS, is that it reduces insulin resistance and the subsequently raised insulin levels that are associated with the condition.[301] As we know, this state of insulin resistance and raised insulin levels increases the risk of other life-threatening conditions like heart disease and type 2 diabetes. It has also been described that there is a low-grade, chronic inflammation associated with PCOS,[302] which as we have learned earlier in the chapter, is implicated in so many different disease processes.

What we have come to understand by now is that a healthy vegan diet can be helpful in all of these problems: obesity, insulin resistance, and inflammation. So can a plant-based diet be helpful for PCOS? Well, the evidence shows that lifestyle interventions that can reduce insulin resistance can also improve outcomes in PCOS, regardless as to whether they result in weight loss or not,[303] and it has been demonstrated that people with PCOS and its related infertility often have an unhealthier diet with fewer whole foods and less fibre,[304, 305] and that these unhealthy diets are associated with more severe symptoms of raised androgens, inflammation and insulin resistance.

There isn't one diet or way of eating that has been recommended in the guidelines for treating PCOS, but some dietary patterns have been shown to be helpful, such as the DASH diet, which is rich in fruits, vegetables, nut and seeds, and has been shown to reduce insulin resistance in PCOS.[306] Whilst we know that a vegan diet has been shown to help with weight loss, in the context of PCOS I could only find one study, which was very small and had a high drop-out rate, and the diet wasn't necessarily useful at helping them maintain weight loss.[307] There aren't many studies which have explored the effects of a vegan diet on PCOS and its associated problems, but it would be logical to presume that it could be beneficial, because we already know that it is useful in treating the associated symptoms and risk factors for PCOS, like insulin resistance, obesity and inflammation, and adherence to the very similar Mediterranean diet can have beneficial effects on androgen levels.[308] It seems that in most dietary interventions, those which are helpful are high in fibre and plant proteins, exerting beneficial effects on the microbiome. That sounds rather like a WFPB diet, doesn't it?

Antibiotic Resistance

Antibiotics are medications that work to kill or reduce the growth of bacteria. You are probably familiar with them because they are frequently prescribed by doctors to treat various common infections, like pneumonia and tonsillitis. In fact, they are prescribed a little too frequently, and antibiotic resistance is becoming a global problem.

Antibiotic resistance describes the way in which infections no longer respond to antibiotics. Microbes have the ability to mutate and change rather rapidly. Think about in-

fluenza and flu vaccines; the reason we need a flu vaccine each year is because the virus mutates, meaning that the previous year's vaccine will no longer work on new strains. In the same way, bacteria mutate and change, but they can do this in response to antibiotics, which put pressure on the bugs to create new strains that will be resistant to the antibiotic, allowing the bacteria to survive.

As a GP, I've been told for many years now that we must be better at antibiotic stewardship by avoiding prescribing antibiotics when they aren't required. No medication should be prescribed unnecessarily, and I couldn't agree more that antibiotics should not be freely prescribed without good evidence that a bacterial infection is present. But what if doctors are being scapegoated, and we're not really the problem? The World Health Organisation (WHO) have described that in some countries, the use of antibiotics in animals exceeds that used in humans.[309] More worryingly, these antibiotics aren't even used solely for the purpose of prevention of infection, which I've discussed in the section on zoonotic disease, but also because low dose antibiotics are useful for their promotion of growth of farmed animals for meat.[310] When there are no new antibiotics in the drug development pipeline, and more multi-drug resistance infections are emerging,[311] how can we continue to allow the animal agriculture industry to continue causing harm to all of us with their use of antibiotics in farmed animals?

Zoonotic Infections

Whilst zoonotic infections aren't necessarily something that we think about as individuals on a day-to-day basis, they are an issue that put us, as part of a global community, at risk. Zoonotic infections are those which can be passed from animals to humans, and of the many examples, there is one that is probably at the forefront of our minds, whether we realise it or not.

COVID-19 is thought to have been zoonotic in origin, with the evidence showing that it likely came from animals, probably from the Wuhan wet-market in China that featured heavily in international news stories when the pandemic broke in 2020. What has stunned me since the pandemic is that despite the public awareness that the captivity, slaughter and sale of animals for human consumption was likely responsible for a terrible infection that affected so many of us, and caused so many deaths, I don't think that people's actions or beliefs about veganism have generally changed. There are, in my opinion, some elements of racism and xenophobia tied up with the views on the origins of COVID, with misguided beliefs that the problem only arose because of the use of animals which we don't really consume in the West. But COVID-19 wasn't a first.

It isn't only 'exotic' meats which are responsible for epidemics and pandemics. Yes, there is some chance that COVID-19 arose from an animal that might not be recognised in the West as food, but there are much wider global practices, which contributed to the outbreak and spread of the disease, and many other infections. In fact, there have been many outbreaks related to the use of more *recognisable-as-food* animals. For example, you have probably heard of avian flu, or 'bird-flu', of which there was a huge outbreak in 2005, leading to the death of 140 million birds, which then went on to spread to humans around the world.[312] And you have must have heard of 'swine-flu', of which there was a significant outbreak in 2009. But MERS (Middle-East respiratory syndrome), SARS (severe-acute respiratory syndrome) and Ebola have all also been associated with the use of animals by humans.

One UN report suggests that 60% of human infections are zoonotic, as are 75% of emerging, or new, infections.[313] The mechanisms for this include the way in which we farm animals; intensive farming puts animals into much more cramped conditions than they would be in nature, increasing their exposure to infections from one another. In addition to this, the animals in herds or flocks have all been bred for a particular set of physical characteristics to ensure they are suitable for purpose: that they will grow fast and provide meat, milk or eggs efficiently. This reduces their genetic diversity which would otherwise have worked towards protecting them from infection, further decreasing their resilience. Another layer to the risk posed to humans from infections that arise in farmed animals is the misuse of antibiotics. One of the purposes may be to prevent outbreaks of infections in the animals, yet the antibiotic resistance which emerges from the widespread use of these drugs is adding fuel to the fire that is zoonotic disease.

Deforestation is a further driver of zoonosis, removing the barriers between humans and animals which then allows pathogens to spill over. We also have to consider the effects of global warming on zoonotic infections; bugs prefer warm environments, so the increasing temperatures we are experiencing globally are encouraging microbial growth. It has also been observed that epidemic zoonoses are often triggered by events such as changes in the climate, floods or famines, and many of these are occurring because of the way in which we are farming animals. It's one great big vicious circle from which we really must step off.

Worryingly, the UN has described that zoonotic infections are increasing in frequency,[314] so whilst following a plant-based diet can improve our individual health, the future wellbeing of the global population also depends upon far less use of animals, and a move towards a plant-based diet.

Global warming and human health

I've covered some of the causes of global warming in the Vegan For The Planet chapter, and discussed why an increase in global temperatures is a concern. Sometimes it's difficult, however, to understand why rising temperatures are harmful to human health. So let's have a quick look at why that might be. Warmer climates result in more cases of infectious diseases, like malaria and zoonotic infections, as well as resulting in a higher risk of malnutrition or starvation due to crop failures. Whole communities can also be displaced in an attempt to avoid the consequent natural disasters that result from global warming, meaning that people can end up in refugee camps, and become at risk from the associated disease that comes with this. Extreme temperatures will be associated with a higher incidence of heat exhaustion and dehydration, both of which are a risk to life. Higher temperatures can also detrimentally affect those with cardiovascular disease, and can increase the risk of pre-diabetes transitioning to type 2 diabetes.

Vegan Take-Aways

A healthy vegan diet is associated with a lower BMI and a reduced risk of obesity, which lowers your risk of many other diseases.

Plant-based diets are associated with a reduced risk of high cholesterol, hypertension, heart disease, dementia, type 2 diabetes, and several cancers.

Removing animal products is beneficial to our health, but addition of healthful ingredients from plants, like polyphenols and phytoestrogens, also confers benefit for many conditions.

Processed meats have been confirmed to cause colon cancer, and red meat probably causes cancer.

Type 2 diabetes has been associated with increased intake of animals proteins.

Around 80% of cases of heart disease could be prevented with lifestyle changes that include eating a healthy diet.

Cholesterol, which is associated with cardiovascular disease, is only found in animal-derived foods. Most saturated fat, which drives the same disease process, is mostly found in animal-derived foods.

Soya protects from the recurrence of breast cancer, the risk of bone fractures in menopause, and reduces menopause symptoms.

Modelling from the data gathered by the EAT-Lancet Commission predicts that the Planetary Health Diet, which is primarily plant-based, could prevent almost 11 million deaths per year.

4

Vegan for Social Justice

'I think there is a connection between . . . the way we treat animals and the way we treat people who are at the bottom of the hierarchy.' —Angela Davis

Ask any vegan, 'Why are you vegan?' and you'll usually hear one of three well known reasons. In fact, they form the titles of the first three chapters of this book; animals, planet, health. I have a personal philosophy that I hope to leave this world just a little better than it was when I came into it. I figured I was working towards this legacy, at first by being vegetarian, and then with my veganism. My feelings that animals deserved equal rights had evolved, and now my veganism extended to the climate and the state of the planet. But I have since come to realise that this still isn't enough. And I don't think I'm alone.

The last couple of years have been particularly difficult, in terms of world politics and social unrest and unease. I feel people have become more aware of the corruption which is rife in the ruling classes, and many are now organising themselves to fight back and be heard. Every week there is a different protest in London. This might be against fossil fuels, or perhaps against the genocide that, as this book is being written, is currently being horrifically wreaked upon the people of Palestine. I feel there's been somewhat of an *'awakening'*.

Let me tell you a bit about my awakening, and no, I'm not just talking about the vegan one I had 9 years ago. I've recently had another, but it's not entirely unconnected; I have started to see the associations between various forms of oppression. Let me give you an example: I went teetotal in 2021. I know, right? Vegan and sober; I promise you I am more fun to hang out with than you might think! I gave up drinking because I realised it had no place in my beautiful life. When I look back, I can now see that its presence dampened and subdued both the great and the sad moments that I've been dealing with throughout my adult life. And despite all the times I involved it in whatever I was doing, it's never given me anything back in return. I take that back. It gave me hangover after hangover. And moderation didn't really work for me, because I am one of those people who doesn't really have an off-switch. If I was pouring a glass of wine, it was unlikely there would be anything left in the bottle the next day. So it had to go.

What has this got to do with veganism or protest, I hear you ask! In my bid to get booze-free, and to maintain it, I turned to the book genre of 'quit-lit'. For those of you who don't know, these are fantastic books written by authors who have been on a similar sobriety journey to help support those of us who are just starting out. Amongst the many great reads, one of my favourites is *Quit Like a Woman* by Holly Whitaker. This book was important because it described the misogyny around the AA movement and sobriety, which was already quite the eye opener – no pun intended. However, I was really stunned when I heard her speaking on a podcast about something she had touched on in the book: that alcohol is used as a tool of oppression. This is done in so many ways, from making the highly addictive substance which is responsible for almost 10,000 deaths in the UK per year[315] readily available at a cost that will profit many members of the ruling class who invest in alcohol companies, to the illegalisation of ceremonial drugs used by indigenous communities, replacing them with the more harmful, but legal, alcohol. I've also read about the corruption of the alcohol industry, with members of the government profiting from alcohol sales, whilst doing little to help the public health cause in reducing the impact of alcohol on human health. Never mind the scant regulation that takes place in the alcohol industry, which is done by itself via Drinkaware.[316] But this is capitalism, isn't it? If money can be made from it, why would the ruling (profiting) classes limit access to it? And if it can be commodified to create wealth, then you can bet your bottom dollar it will be.

(As a side note, I think it was this idea of the greater, insidious harms of alcohol, and its use to oppress that really spurred me on to remain sober, more than the idea of preventing harm to myself. I sometimes think this ability to commit for reasons greater than my own wellbeing stemmed, in part, from my experiences and journey with veganism. People who have dabbled in veganism and given up have often been vegan for their own health or benefit, whereas those who have chosen to live vegan for the planet or animals often report finding it easier to remain committed, because there is more at stake. There is a greater good.)

This association that was made between alcohol and oppression opened up a whole world of ideas for me. I began to make connections between so much of what we're taking part in every day, and systemic oppression and racism. I saw this being further explored by Dr Chris Van Tulleken in his book *Ultra-Processed People*, where he described the displacement of indigenous people from their homes because of land clearance for agriculture and food production.[317] The more I read about the food industry, the more sure I am that the only way to kick back at the establishment, with more than just protest and non-violent direct action, is to be careful about what we consume, and where we spend our money. And I'm pretty sure that veganism is a very good starting point for rejecting some of these norms. Let me explain why.

Anti-Colonialism/Anti-Racism

Land use

Chris Van Tulleken, in his book *Ultra-Processed People*, describes modern-day colonial acts that involve displacement of indigenous peoples. Sadly, displacement happens for so many different, unjustified reasons, but the context in which Dr Van Tulleken discusses it is in the production of ultra-processed foods (UPFs). But dig a little deeper and you'll see that while this is a huge issue, so is that of livestock production, which I've also described in the 'Vegan for the Planet' chapter. Land clearance and deforestation damages the environment and contributes negatively to climate change, but the practice also harms indigenous communities. It displaces them, removing their homes, sources of food and livelihoods, and sometimes even directly results in their deaths. Global Witness have described violence against indigenous people defending their land from those trying to take it by force for various reasons, including industrial logging, mining and farming.[318] Globally, there were 342 killings between 2012 and 2021, with 50 of those victims being small-scale farmers.

Indigenous communities often take on the role of protecting the land, still having a close relationship with the environment because of their reliance on it for food, shelter and livelihood. They are still very much connected to the land, acting as custodians of it. And, amongst other culprits, the animal agriculture industry is having a direct effect on them. The *Guardian* published a report about one indigenous community whose land in South America has been un-lawfully taken and used to breed cattle for beef.[319] This has affected their ability to fish and hunt for their own foods, as well as poison-ing their crops with pesticides. Much of the beef produced by the company who is farming on that land is used by Western companies such as Nestlé, McDonalds and Burger King. Greenpeace reports a similar story, describing how the global meat industry has resulted in land being stolen from indigenous Brazilian communities as defor-estation for animal grazing continues.[320] And even if this land isn't used specifically for breeding cattle for beef, it is often used to grow the soya used to feed them. Not, as avid carnivores would have you believe, grown to feed solely vegans; around 80% of all soya is used in livestock feed, whilst humans only consume around 7%.[321]

These injustices against indigenous communities are further ex-aggerated when we consider that they are often the first to be im-pacted by the effects of global warming, too. Despite making up just 5% of the world's population, they look after 20–25% of the earth's land surface[322] – land which holds 80% of the earth's biodi-versity. Due to climate change, they are at more risk of disease asso-ciated with rising temperatures, drought and forest fires, damage to seedlings and crops because of excessive rainfall, and worsening food insecurity because of changes to endemic insect life.

Isn't it always the most vulnerable that are the most hard hit by the escalating effects of capitalism and its sequelae though?

Lactose intolerance

Doesn't it seem odd that I'm naming lactose intolerance as being as-sociated with colonialism and racism? But hear me out. Whilst milk has previously been co-opted as a symbol of white nationalism for the rather obvious reason of its appearance,[323] even the marketing of milk as a universally healthy product could also be deemed racist. The whole reason behind this is the issue of lactose intolerance, and who it affects.

I'm often amazed by the conviction with which people who are lactose intolerant attempt to continue consuming dairy. I have had patients request a prescription for lactase (see below for more on this) in order to enable them to continue drinking milk and eating cheese. The supermarkets' 'free from' fridges always contain lactose-free options right next to the plant milks, further demonstrating this inexplicable desire for dairy. I find it really hard to fathom why the lactose intolerant don't just switch to plant milks and cheeses instead, especially when product quality has improved so much, and the nutrient content is often fairly comparable, by design, and the harmful effects of dairy can be completely avoided. But it's scenarios like these which demonstrate just how much we've been convinced by the dairy industry that we need to continue consuming cow's milk products. But how is this, in and of itself, racist?

Well, did you know that 65% of the world's population is lactose intolerant?[324] And most of those affected by lactose intolerance are black and global majority people? For example, in Northern European countries, the prevalence of lactose intolerance can be as low as 2%.[325] But in the US, a more ethnically diverse country, the distribution of lactose maldigestion is as follows: 79% of Native Americans, 75% of black people, 51% of Hispanic people, and 21% of Caucasians.[326] For a product that is indigestible by the global majority to be pushed so hard as a healthy foodstuff, so convincingly that people request medication in order to be able to consume it, despite it being actually unnecessary and harmful to humans, the planet, and cows, just speaks to the agenda of putting profit over health and ethics by a racist, profiteering dairy industry.

The absurdity of how dairy has been put so firmly into our dietary recommendations and guidelines is particularly apparent when one considers the function of lactase, the enzyme which is deficient in those who are lactose intolerant. Lactose is a sugar found in milk. It is broken down by the enzyme lactase, and as you would expect, most newborns have high levels of lactase, and it then declines after weaning. It is thought that our ancestors probably started out as lactose intolerant, but then some populations developed a genetic mutation leading to lactase persistence, which allowed them to continue consuming a product meant for babies and infants. So, our natural state as humans was that we didn't consume the milk of another animal. But honestly, does this really need to be stated? It seems rather obvious to me.

Cow's milk is unnecessary to human health, and even if we accept the fact that many of us might be able to consume dairy, we absolutely have the choice to replace this with equally nutritious, and less environmentally harmful products like oat and soya milk, and cheeses made from fermented, blended cashews.

Animal processing plants

Greenpeace has described how the industrial meat system is responsible for serious crimes against humans.[327] In a report on the violence behind the meat industry, they describe that in Germany, 80% of those employed in meat packing facilities are poorly treated migrants, and that human trafficking and mistreatment of employees is rife. Much of this was exposed during the COVID pandemic, and a European report looking into COVID outbreaks in meat processing facilities found that migrant workers were often earning 40–50% less than regular staff.[328]

In the US, African-Americans have been disproportionately affected by the unpleasant conditions associated with living near industrial pig farms, a situation described as environmental racism.[329] Stories are emerging about people whose families have lived on their land for generations, now being exposed to sickening smells and the increased infection risk associated with waste lagoons on these farms.[330] As we've already heard, these lagoons are pools of pig faeces. Whilst animal processing plants are, for obvious reasons, built in rural areas out of the view of the general population, they are often placed on land inhabited primarily by people of colour, who are therefore disproportionately affected by these unpleasant settings.

Feminism

I once wrote an article about an episode of *The Handmaid's Tale*, and what I thought were subtle messages it contained about the similarities between the fate of the handmaids and that of dairy cows.[331] To those who haven't yet made the connection, this might seem farfetched. But, to those of us who have made the transition to veganism *and* who identify as feminist the links are as clear as day. For anybody who hasn't read the book or watched the TV show, which is rather brilliant and based on the fantastic book by Margaret Atwood, it is set in a dystopian world in which humans are mostly infertile. There is a ruling class of patriarchs, who run a totalitarian political system in which women are all subservient. Those who were able to conceive just prior to the collapse of society are captured and kept as handmaids: women who are assigned to the households of the wealthy commanders in order to become impregnated by them, providing them and their wives with a child, before being moved onto the next house for their next assignment.

The similarities I have drawn between the handmaids and dairy cows include the commodification of their reproductive organs, the removal of their young as if they are not their own, the loss of autonomy over their own bodies, and the brutalisation they are subjected to if they don't submit to all of the cruelties done to them. In this particular episode which I wrote about, the main character, a handmaid called Offred, finds herself floating in the dark in a large tank of milk during an escape bid. The images were stark and striking; and rather symbolic, I feel.

Most animals don't have a gender, as such, but might have sexual characteristics that identify them as male or female, such as a large set of antlers, a colourful plumage, or a mane. Beyond reproduction, their sex doesn't really matter at all in the natural world, but in the same way that a binary gender system has been enforced upon us in our modern, capitalist hell, animals that are utilised by humans are also sexed or gendered by us. I've already touched on this in the animal rights chapter, where I discuss the fate of the dairy cow, or the hen and her male chicks. I've described it in the context of the cruel fates of these animals, but when we consider that female cows are so abused and tortured because of their femaleness, I can't help but think that feminists should be up in arms about the commodification of the female body of any animal.

The use and abuse of the female cow's body also extends to her motherhood. Not only is she regularly assaulted to make her pregnant, but once she gives birth, her infant is taken from her. I've seen video after video of mothers running after a trailer containing her newborn calf. It's just heartbreaking. But it's also anger inducing. The audacity of these (mostly) male farmers, forcing their fists into the back passage of female cows during the insemination process, removing their young, then stealing their precious milk is sickening to me. As is putting her through this over, and over, and over again until she is physically exhausted and then slaughtered. My journey through veganism keeps bringing me back to *connections*. In abusing animals in this way, not only are we forgetting our connection with our non-human neighbours on this planet, and with the natural earth, having lost all respect for them, but we're also depriving other animals of their connection with their young. This is probably one of the only things that matter to them, beyond their own survival. But we're also taking that, aren't we?

The female chicken is also exploited because of her 'gender'. And I have questioned the use of the word gender versus sex here too, but again, this feels like a situation where a binary gender system has been forced upon these animals for a purpose. Hens in the wild would be producing far fewer eggs than they do in captivity. But industrial egg production forces her to produce a disproportionately large amount, putting her health at risk. Not only does her sex force her to risk her own health and physical comfort for a process that has been unnaturally manipulated, but it also forces her into a life of captivity, beak clipping and, again, deprivation of the connection of motherhood.

It's not just cows and chickens who are deprived of the experience to mother as nature intended. If you've ever seen the conditions in which sows are kept during pregnancy and early motherhood, I'm sure you've been horrified. I first witnessed this on a school trip to a university farm. I have strong memories of an overwhelming smell of manure filling my nostrils, while I climbed on a metal fence to peer over at a pink, plump creature lying on her side. I could see that the pig I was watching wasn't able to stand, and I felt sad for her, but I didn't fully understand why this was happening. Now I know she was in a farrowing crate, a metal contraption designed to keep a pregnant pig lying on her side, where she will stay until her piglets are born and weaned off her milk. Farmers will tell you that this is to keep her piglets safe; to prevent her from rolling over onto them. But I'm sure they are describing a sad side effect of farming, because I don't think that pigs with all the space of a wild environment have an endemic problem of rolling over onto their young. I also wonder whether the welfare of piglets is really what is at stake here, or rather the potential loss of product and profit.

When we consider the connections between us and our non-human neighbours, the overlaps of our rights and our needs bear more similarities than differences. This is why I've come to describe myself as an intersectional vegan, but I'll write more about this shortly. And it's not just in the similarities between human and non-human female animals that we can see why the causes of feminism and veganism intersect. We've already seen how a plant-rich life can be better for the environment, and there is evidence that climate change disproportionately affects women's health.[332] I don't think I will ever stop being amazed at the connections between us and the natural world.

Anti-Capitalism

As with water, electricity, and even health care, food has been turned into a commodity to be bought and sold. What a sad, sick situation, that our basic human needs can be withheld unless we have the means to buy them, whilst making others wealthier than any person ought to be. I'm not sure that veganism would have become such a strong, necessary movement if it wasn't for factory farming, the shocking birth-child of capitalism and animal agriculture. There is, perhaps, some argument that consuming animal products has been a natural part of human evolution. We are, by nature, omnivores, after all. I could argue from a philosophical point about how in some parts of the world, we now have the ability and capacity to make dif-

ferent decisions about what we eat than our ancestors, or of communities in parts of the world with no choice but to consume animal
products. But now that the human population has been growing
out of control, the demand for meat, dairy and eggs could only have
been met by a vast animal agriculture industry which farms animals
to an unfathomable scale. Of course there will always be somebody
willing and happy to provide the product which is being demanded.
And the cost isn't just monetary.

The agricultural revolution was the start of what we see today
of the industrial animal farming system. With it came the domesti-
cation of large animals, and the beginning of their ongoing era of
misery. Karl Marx said, 'At the core of the capitalist system . . . lies
the complete separation of the consumer from the means of production'.[333] And, oh, how this applies to the animal agriculture industry.
It has been argued that the 'animal agriculture industry exemplifies
Marx's theory of objectification inherent in capitalism, commodi-
fying non-human animals as "an external object, a thing through
which its qualities satisfies human needs of whatever kind."'[334]

I also argue that it's not just the non-human animals which are
commodified, but also people who are working within the animal
processing system. Imagine going to work every day where the only
task you'll have is to slaughter, over and over, until it's going-home
time. Imagine spending your whole day around animals who are full
of stress and fear, sometimes making eye contact with them in their
last moments on this earth. Imagine being the one to slice the knife
across their throats, or press the button that dunks them into the
boiling water when they might not be dead yet, or to throw the male
chicks down a chute to their death. Imagine knowing that you're responsible for hundreds or thousands of deaths. So, it is no wonder
that abattoir workers suffer from an increased risk of PTSD (post-
traumatic stress disorder), and another condition known as perpe-

tration-induced traumatic stress (PITS).[335] The psychological stress that slaughterhouse workers are put under can also lead to increased crime and violent behaviours,[336] and when we consider the following experience of an abattoir worker, it's really not that surprising:

'Whether they eat meat or not, most people in the UK have never been inside an abattoir – and for good reason. They are filthy, dirty places. There's animal faeces on the floor, you see and smell the guts, and the walls are covered in blood . . . As I spent day after day in that large, windowless box, my chest felt increasingly heavy and a grey fog descended over me. At night, my mind would taunt me with nightmares, replaying some of the horrors I'd witnessed throughout the day.'[337]

In the US, it has been documented that meat packing is one of the most dangerous jobs, with the rate of injury more than twice that of the national average.[338] And as we've already seen, it is yet again, the most vulnerable of society that are affected the most badly:

'The workers, most often immigrants and resettled refugees, slaughter and process hundreds of animals an hour, forced to work at high speeds in cold conditions, doing thousands of the same repetitions over and over, with few breaks.'[339]

All of this violence, harm and exploitation, when the alternative is more nutritious and less harmful to the environment, is justified because of the profit it makes. This is only one tiny part of the capitalist picture. But when the lives and health of vulnerable people that are so dreadfully affected, as well as the non-human victims caught up in the industry, how can we continue to excuse it?

World Hunger

Globally, more than 820 million people remain undernourished[340] and, worryingly, our population continues to rise. Earth's population is estimated to reach 10 billion by 2050. That's really not very long. The ruling classes, who undoubtedly, will always remain well-fed, would have you believe that this is a population issue, not a food one. Yes, the world's population is huge; at the time of writing this book, it is around 8 billion. That's a lot of mouths to feed! But you'll realise how nonsensical it is to feed this population animal protein when you consider that you also need to feed the 82 billion animals that are farmed and slaughtered every year in order to do this. Livestock are fed 41% of the world's grains, but if we used the land on which this is grown to farm crops for human consumption, we could feed an additional 3.5 billion people.[341] It is estimated that livestock consume five times more food than the entire human population of Earth, so why don't we start feeding this to the planet's human population, instead, and put an end to world hunger? The rich can do without their steak, and we'll all benefit from removing unhealthy animal proteins from our diet.

When you consider these figures, the EAT-Lancet commission just makes more and more sense. I wrote about it in the 'Vegan For Health' chapter, but to recap, it was led by scientists from around the world, to work out how we feed a growing population of humans a healthy diet, which is sustainable within planetary boundaries. As part of their research, one of their biggest considerations was famine, and the huge number of people around the world who go hungry. When we can solve world hunger, improve human health, reduce the impact of our farming practices on the environment AND reduce suffering to animals, veganism really does seem like the only sensible option.

Total Liberation

Total liberation is 'a political philosophy and movement that combines anarchism with a commitment to animal and earth liberation'.[342] It basically covers much of what we've already discussed: it's anticapitalism, it's anti-oppression, it's for animal rights, human rights, LGBTQ+ rights, and against the assault on the environment. It is a way of understanding how all forms of oppression are connected, and how to fight against them.

When the civil rights leader Fannie Lou Hamer said 'nobody is free until everybody's free',[343] she was referring to the intersection between racism and feminism, imploring white women to recognise the damage being done by the white patriarchy. Intersectionality is a framework for understanding how the identities of different groups of individuals overlap to result in many different positions of both privilege and disadvantage; for example, the world experience of a white woman will be very different of that of a black woman, whose experiences would be different again from an Asian trans woman. We are not identified by just one of our traits, but are rather a jumble of identities and experiences. Which is why it is important to acknowledge that there isn't just one cause that is important; white feminists should be anti-racist to support their sisters around the globe; all feminists should be supportive of LGBTQ+ rights to include their sisters who weren't born female; all feminists should consider the rights of female animals used and abused for their reproductive organs and abilities, living a kinder, vegan life.

Intersectional veganism extends our principles to include all victims of oppression. So whilst we're fighting for the rights of animals, we're also raising our voices for humans who are oppressed because of their skin colour, or their 'class', or sexuality, or gender. Because these things are all connected. And with that, the oppression overlaps with capitalism and its victims, the destruction of the natural world, health inequalities, and world hunger. This is why I believe that total liberation is the ultimate fight against all that is wrong in the world. But veganism done well is a great place to start.

Vegan Take-Aways

Animal processing plants, and the meat industry in general, disproportionately affect minority groups, meaning that it isn't just non-human animals that are the victims in the meat industry.

Nobody is free until everybody is free. Hhow can you believe that non-human animals should be free, whilst ignoring the oppression of other people?

Agriculture, predominantly animal agriculture, displaces indigenous communities.

Dairy is advertised as a healthful food, despite a global majority being lactose intolerant.

World hunger could be solved if we ate the crops we grow instead of feeding them to farmed animals destined for the food industry.

STAYING WELL

So, you've read all about why we should all consider following a plant-rich life, but now you need to know where to start. Or maybe you're worried about how to do this well, and how to maintain health.

Let me help you. This section will tell you what you need to know about the basics of nutrition, and how a vegan diet can affect that. So read on to find out what you might need to consider.

5

Protein

What is it and why do I need it?

Proteins are long chain molecules which are the building blocks of all living things. Every one of our cells, all of our hormones and secretions, and the enzymes which help all of our daily processes that keep us alive are all made from proteins. And, whilst they provide 4kcal of energy for every 1g, helping to fuel us and making up around 10–15% of our dietary energy, their key role in our diet is for growth, repair and maintenance of the body's tissues, such as muscle.

As I've already mentioned, protein is required for many different roles, from comprising the structure of our bodies, to moving micronutrients from one cell to another, and composing the antibodies that fight infection. Proteins can be further broken down into peptides, which are made up by amino acids. There are 9 'essential' amino acids, which need to be obtained from the diet, as we are unable to make these within the human body. Although conventionally thought of as being found in meats, amino acids, and as such protein, can be found in all plant-based foods.

What's 'normal'?

The current recommendation for intake of protein is 0.75g for every kg of body weight, per day. This equates to around 45g of protein per day for the average woman, and 56g for the average man. But in the UK, the average woman eats around 67g of protein every day, while the average man eats 85g,[344] more than we actually require. There is some thought that plant-based protein might not be absorbed quite as well as animal proteins because of the higher fibre content, and it's because of this that Plant Based Health Professionals UK, a trusted source of information for vegans and healthcare professionals alike, settle on a recommended intake of 1g of protein for every kg of body weight.[345] And we must remember that the fibre that plant proteins come with, whilst it reduces the amount of protein absorbed, adds a wealth of other health benefits. If we aim for 1g of protein per kg of weight, our intake would still be lower than that which most people in the UK consume, but higher than official guidelines advise. This is all very achievable as long as we are reaching our energy requirements and varying our protein sources.

There are situations where requirements might differ, however, for example if you are pregnant or breast(/chest)feeding, or an athlete, in which case you might need to tailor your protein intake accordingly. There has been some contention about our protein requirements as we age, too; some sources state that we need more as we get older,[346] but others, including Dr Greger of Nutrition Facts, suggest that protein restriction is better for aging.[347] Plant Based Health Professionals UK recommend that older adults aim for an intake of 1.2–1.6g of plant protein per kg of bodyweight to maintain health and avoid the bone and muscle loss that can occur with ageing.

What happens if I don't have enough?

It's quite difficult to not achieve the recommended daily intake of protein, particularly when eating a well varied diet of whole foods, fruits, vegetables, pulses and seeds, as they are all made up of amino acids. There used to be a common misbelief that some of the essential amino acids couldn't be obtained without consuming meat; however, as long as your intake of plant-based proteins is plenty and varied, there should be no concern.

A protein deficiency would probably only be seen as part of a picture of general malnutrition, in somebody who is in a starvation state, rather than somebody with dietary restrictions. As such there aren't any tests to ensure one is consuming enough protein, but in clinical scenarios where nutritional status needs to be checked, blood albumin levels are sometimes used. These are not very reliable, however, and I wouldn't be checking the albumin level of most of my patients for this indication.

Where can vegans find it?

Protein is found in all plant-based foods, but some are better sources than others. Chickpeas contain around 8g of protein per 100g when cooked, whilst whole grains like oats, quinoa and wholewheat flour contain around 12g of protein per 100g. However products like tofu and tempeh which are products made from soya beans can contain anywhere between 10 and 20g per 100g respectively. It has been a long held belief that plant proteins are incomplete, meaning they are lacking in certain essential amino acids, however all plant foods contain all essential amino acids, just in varying amounts. Beans and legumes tend to contain less methionine whilst grains contain less lysine, however if you eat enough and vary your sources throughout the day, this difference does not matter. It's also important to note that you also do not need to specifically combine sources at the same meal either, contrary to some schools of thought.

The bonus of getting all your protein from plants is that you simultaneously consume fibre which is great for the gut and heart, and you avoid all of the saturated fat and cholesterol that is associated with animal proteins.

6

Fats

What is it and why do I need it?

Fats are the richest source of calories of all the macronutrients, with 1g providing 9kcal of energy. They are made up of fatty acids, the building blocks of fat, which can be saturated or unsaturated. This description is related to how many hydrogen atoms are attached to it, but in simple (and important) terms, saturated fats are generally not good for human health, whereas unsaturated, polyunsaturated and monounsaturated fats are better. There is, however, a kind of unsaturated fat called 'trans' fat, which can occur naturally in some red meat and dairy, and this is usually found in hydrogenated vegetable oils. Trans fats are detrimental to health and there have been public health measures to reduce the amount of these found in foods.

Healthy fats, however, are a very important part of human nutrition, and it is recommended that they should make up 35% of our diet. As well as providing energy, they assist with the absorption of the fat-soluble vitamins A, D, E and K, and are used in the structure of cell walls, and even within cells for important reactions. Most fats can be made within the human body from the building blocks, fatty acids, but as with the amino acids, there are some which are 'essential' meaning that they need to be obtained in the diet. Now this is where the vegan diet could start to become deficient if it isn't well planned, as the two essential fatty acids are omega-3 and omega-6, for which fish, meat and eggs are often relied upon as sources.

What's 'normal'?

The recommended daily intake of fat is 70g for women, and 95g for men, with no more than 20g and 30g respectively of this being saturated fat. Recommendations also advise that fat intake should be no more than 35% of your total energy consumption, and saturated fat no more than 11%. Intakes in the UK are currently close to these recommendations, but saturated fats are slightly up at 12% of the average intake.

What happens if I don't have enough?

Fats are another component of the diet that we don't really measure in everyday medical practice. We do, however, measure parameters like cholesterol and triglycerides, which can cause poor health when they are raised. But because we don't have measures for 'normal' fat levels in the body, it is difficult to know when you might be deficient. There are private clinics who use tests to measure your omega-3 levels, but I've never seen this done in the NHS. Dietary omega fatty acids have been associated with improved cardiovascular health, are important in child development, and have been implicated in reducing the risk of Alzheimer's disease,[348] although the evidence for these benefits is not particularly strong.

Where can vegans find it?

Many people rely on meat and dairy for dietary fats. However these are often saturated, which, as we've discussed, can be related to a higher risk of several health problems such as heart disease. Most plant-based fats are not saturated, with the exception of coconut and palm oil, which should only be consumed sparingly, if at all. Vegan sources of fats include nuts, seeds and avocados, and when consumed whole, these are all particularly healthy. It is when these foods are processed into oils that the health benefits are reduced, but the bottom line is that they are still better for you than their animal-derived counterparts.

It's also easy to get tripped up with balancing the essential fats. Although most omegas come from fish, eggs and meat, there are plenty of vegan sources of these, such as rapeseed oil, walnuts, chia, flax and hemp seeds for omega-3, and sunflower oil, avocado and peanut butter for omega-6. But while these sources are readily found, we need to consider the ratio of omega-3 to omega-6. If too much omega-6 is consumed, we don't convert omega-3s to their useful components particularly well, and this reduces the amount of these omega-3s in our blood. The simplest way around this is to keep a balanced intake of plant-based fats, forget about omega-6, as it's likely you're getting plenty, and consciously increase your intake of omega-3 rich foods, or take a daily DHA and EPA supplement.

DHA, or docosahexaenoic acid, and EPA, or eicosapentaenoic acid, are two of the omega-3 fatty acids and are often converted from the third, alpha-linolenic acid (ALA). The conversion rates of ALA to DHA and EPA is inefficient, which means that consuming DHA and EPA directly is recommended. Unfortunately, these are usually found in fish, meaning that it's difficult for vegans to obtain these nutrients directly. So, although we can find plenty of ALA in plant-based foods, we can't always guarantee a good conversion rate of this

to the really important DHA and EPA. This is the reason why I recommend a supplement of vegan DHA and EPA, but also ensuring
you eat plenty of flaxseeds, as well as other dietary omega-3 sources.

7

Carbohydrates

What is it and why do I need it?

Carbohydrates are the main source of energy in the human diet, and should make up 50% of our energy intake. There are 3 main types of carbohydrate: starchy carbohydrates, sugars and dietary fibre. Sugars and starches provide 3.75kcal/g of energy to the body's tissues, which require a constant supply of glucose. If this supply isn't met with carbohydrates, glucose can be made from the two other macronutrients: protein and fat. However, if enough calories are not consumed from any of the three macronutrients, then malnutrition may occur.

Dietary fibre, or resistant starch, isn't relied on by the body for energy, and it is not digested or absorbed in the small intestine. However, when it reaches the large intestine, it is fermented and metabolised by the bacteria living in the colon, the microbiome we've already heard so much about, which does produce a small amount of energy, at around 2kcal/g. But just because it doesn't necessarily provide us with energy, it doesn't mean that fibre isn't super important. For years, we've been underestimating the value of dietary fibre, particularly for the health of parts of our anatomy other than the gut, such as the cardiovascular system. But as you will have read in the 'Vegan for Health' chapter, we are now beginning to understand that fibre is really important in maintaining a healthy microbiome, and thus impacting many other facets of our health.

What's 'normal'?

The daily reference intake of carbohydrates for adults is 260g per day, and the Eatwell guide suggests that one third of our diet should be made up from starchy foods such as potatoes, rice and pasta, which are rich in carbohydrates. To make sure that you are reaping the benefits of other aspects of carbohydrates, make sure to aim for wholegrain versions of these foods.

What happens if I don't have enough?

If we don't get enough carbohydrates in our diet, blood sugar levels can drop, causing hypoglycaemia. This can make you feel a bit unwell, with light-headedness, nausea or sweating. But our bodies are very good at switching to utilise other sources of energy, such as protein and fat, as fuel. This isn't necessarily a bad thing, but if you don't have many resources in terms of body fat, then you might struggle with tiredness and low energy if you're not eating enough carbohydrates. You may even lose weight, but as some people choose to follow a 'low-carb' diet for this reason, it can be helpful in certain situations.

A major downside of not consuming enough carbohydrates is that you would be at risk of not eating enough fibre. As I mentioned above, fibre is such an important part of our diet, and can't be found without eating carbohydrates.

Where can vegans find it?

Sugars can be intrinsic, which means they are in the cellular structure of the food, as with vegetables and fruits, or extrinsic such as in juices and processed sugars. The rest of the carbohydrates are classified as 'complex', and this includes the starches and fibre. Starchy carbohydrates are found in potatoes, bread, rice and pasta. Dietary fibre or resistant starch is found in many plant foods such as fruits, vegetables, grains and beans.

8

Iron

What is it and why do I need it?

Iron is one of those micronutrients that seems to cause vegans (and non-vegans) more concern than others. When your iron level is low, it can cause a condition called anaemia which can be explained as the state of low haemoglobin levels in the blood. But what is iron? And, while we're at it, what is haemoglobin?

Haemoglobin, often shortened to Hb, is a protein found in red blood cells which carry oxygen around the body. It's a pretty important little protein, as oxygen is needed by every one of our cells in order to function. Iron is a mineral nutrient which is a vital component of the Hb molecule, mainly because it's the part which actually bonds with oxygen, picking it up in the lungs and carrying it around the body.

What's 'normal'?

Whilst iron levels can be measured directly with a blood test, doctors often measure another parameter, a protein called 'ferritin'. Ferritin carries iron around the body in your blood, and so it can be a reliable measure of your actual iron levels. Ferritin levels of less than

30mcg/L indicate iron deficiency, but, in practice, I have found that many people feel quite tired and under the weather when their ferritin levels are below 60mcg/L. Measurements of both iron and ferritin levels are quite complex, because numbers above the top end of the reference range can also be problematic, but don't always relate to a high intake of iron-rich foods. In fact, a raised ferritin can be caused by completely non-food related diseases, and can be a marker of inflammation.

A low iron level will initially cause your red blood cells to reduce in size, a state known as microcytosis (you may hear your doctor mention this if you have been diagnosed with anaemia). This is one of the signs those clever blood analysis machines look for in the diagnosis of iron deficiency anaemia. A person can have low iron levels without being anaemic, but in all likelihood, if this iron isn't replaced they would become anaemic after the cells have begun shrinking down and become microcytic.

When we talk about 'blood count', what we're usually referring to is the value for haemoglobin. The ranges for normal haemoglobin also vary between males and females, and anaemia is a Hb of less than 120g/L in women who aren't pregnant, less than 110g/L in pregnant women, and less than 130g/L in men. There are lots of causes of anaemia, but I'll cover the dietary ones here.

Now, just to complicate matters, iron isn't the only nutrient which causes anaemia when we run low on it. I won't discuss it in this chapter, but vitamin B12 deficiency can also cause anaemia, and so can a low folic acid level. But, back to iron! There are also medical conditions which can reduce your iron level, resulting in anaemia, but for the sake of simplicity, and keeping it relevant to our topic here, we'll assume that when I'm writing about iron deficiency, it's because of decreased dietary intake.

What happens if I don't have enough?

I think it's quite clear now that if you are not getting enough iron in your diet, you may be at risk of becoming anaemic. People who menstruate are particularly at risk of this, because as previously mentioned, when you have a regular period you lose blood, and therefore iron, every month. Pregnant people also become anaemic much more easily, as their bodies are trying to make blood cells at a quicker rate so their baby is also well supplied, and there may not be an adequate enough iron intake to keep up with this.

The most common symptom of anaemia is tiredness. Unfortunately this is a very vague symptom which is also caused by many other conditions, but if you are at risk of anaemia (vegans could be at risk, particularly young, menstruating vegans) and feel more tired than usual, it could be worth considering anaemia as a potential cause. Other symptoms include headaches, a sore tongue, or cracking at the corners of the mouth, and hair thinning. Again, some of these are nonspecific, in that they can be caused by other conditions or deficiencies.

More serious symptoms which could indicate severe anaemia are shortness of breath, particularly when exerting yourself – for example, climbing the stairs or walking uphill – and chest pain or palpitations, again particularly when exerting yourself. There are also signs which your doctor may look for when they examine you, and these include spoon-shaped nails, your skin or the inside of your eyes looking pale, and a fast heart rate (tachycardia).

If anaemia is left untreated and becomes severe, it can cause more serious problems. You may become more prone to catching infections and your heart could start to struggle with pumping effectively if the anaemia is severe enough. It is unusual to develop such severe anaemia from a deficiency in your diet, but any of these symptoms should be investigated by your doctor.

Your GP will be able to examine you and arrange a full blood count and iron level to determine if you are deficient in iron and if you have become anaemic. Unfortunately, many of the iron supplements which are available for you to buy do not have a high enough dose of iron in them, so depending on how severe the iron deficiency or anaemia is, you may have to take prescribed iron for a short time, and then you may be able to get back onto a shop-bought, vegan supplement or incorporating more iron-rich foods into your diet. Your GP will be able to advise you more about what you might require.

Where can vegans find it?

The recommended daily intake of iron is 14.8mg for women aged less than 50, and 8.7mg for women over 50 and men. But, this is the amount required to stay healthy, not the amount required in somebody who already has low iron levels. Iron is found in many foods, and many people would think of meat and liver as iron-rich foods, but there are plenty of sources where vegans can get their iron. For example, did you know that lentils contain around the same amount of iron as beef, weight for weight?

It is worth noting that there are two types of iron found in the diet. The type we get from plant-based foods, non-haem iron, is absorbed slightly differently than the haem iron found in meats, and unfortunately, is not absorbed quite as well. This is mainly because the structure of the iron molecule is slightly different, and needs to be changed by our stomachs before it can be absorbed, but this can be interfered with by other things we are consuming. For example, the tannins in tea or a lot of fibre can stop us absorbing our plant-based iron efficiently. However, taking it with a vitamin C source, such as orange juice can actually enhance its absorption, or you could consider having fruit rich in vitamin C for dessert, or a side salad containing tomatoes. If you have read the chapter 'Vegan for Health', you've probably got the gist by now that non-haem iron is the healthier option over all, despite being the harder to absorb, because it bypasses all of the harmful side effects of haem iron.

I've already mentioned that lentils are a great source of iron, but so are quinoa, chickpeas and beans, including soya and even tinned baked beans! As Popeye was well aware, dark green leafy vegetables like spinach contain a good amount of iron, and so do kale and peas. There are some great iron-rich snacks too, including nuts such as almonds and pistachios, as well as dried fruits like raisins and apricots. Even tinned fruits like blackcurrants, raspberries and cherries can be a good iron source, as well as canned coconut milk. Apart from the whole foods I have written about, lots of processed foods are fortified with iron too, as are cereals; pasta and bread can also be a great source.

There are plenty of good sources of iron in the vegan diet, but if you are worried about your intake, there are multivitamins which contain iron. For example, health food shops usually sell a vegan multivitamin which contains much of your recommended daily dose of iron, or alternatively just a pure iron supplement. But as most of the iron rich, plant-based foods contain many other nutrients (as well as being super tasty), it's very easy to get what you need by just munching on some great vegan food.

9

Calcium

What is it and why do I need it?

Calcium is a mineral which is needed for many processes within the human body. Most people know that it's used to make bone, and in the same vein, it's also involved in keeping teeth healthy. But did you know it's also essential for healthy blood clotting, normal muscle and nerve activity, and even for helping our chromosomes move when our cells need to divide?

What's 'normal'?

The range for calcium differs depending on the laboratory doing the testing, but a normal level is usually quoted as being between 2.05 and 2.60 mmol/l. This is the 'corrected calcium' level, which just means that the level of the protein albumin in circulating blood is also taken into consideration, as calcium binds to albumin in order to move around the body.

Blood tests for calcium levels are not very useful for day-to-day monitoring. The reason for this is that our bodies regulate our calcium level by moving it in and out of bone, which essentially act as a calcium store. This means that it is difficult to know if we are getting enough, as you may be taking far less calcium than is recommended, but your blood test may show normal levels. When your blood calcium levels drop, hormones are released which encourage bone to release calcium into the bloodstream, and when it's too high, the bones reabsorb some.

What happens if I don't have enough?

There are certain medical conditions which can severely alter your calcium levels, and this is usually when an abnormal result is picked up. But more often than not, doctors will suspect that you could require more calcium in your diet if an x-ray picks up that your bones are a little thinner than they should be, which is called osteopenia.

In the medical conditions which do cause serious calcium level abnormalities, when your levels are low, you can suffer from cramping and tingling in the hands or feet, fits and psychiatric problems. As I previously mentioned, it's extremely unlikely you would get a deficiency to this extent from not having adequate dietary intake. It would be more likely that you got a diagnosis of osteopenia or osteoporosis (low bone density) after having an x-ray or breaking bones in an unexpected manner. So, as you can see, testing for calcium levels is not very useful, and it is far more important to just maintain a healthy intake. If you are unsure that you take enough calcium in your diet, there is a brilliant online calculator which can be found at www.osteoporosis.foundation.

Where can vegans find it?

We're all used to seeing adverts for dairy as a good source of calcium, but there are plenty of ways in which vegans can top up too. For example, enriched soya milk contains the same amount of calcium as dairy milk: 240mg per 200ml. Tofu is also a great source when it is 'calcium-set', which many in the UK are, containing up to 500mg of calcium per 100g. To be sure it is calcium-set, look for calcium sulphate in the ingredient list. Other foods with high calcium content are white beans, spinach, figs, Brazil nuts, apricots and chickpeas.

The recommended daily intake is around 800mg; however, people who are pregnant or breast(/chest)feeding need 50% more than that, and teenagers do, too.

Calcium supplements are often taken with vitamin D, and this is because the two of them work synergistically to keep our bones healthy. Vitamin D enhances the absorption of calcium from the gut and increases the amount that is laid down in bone. Vitamin D levels can be easily checked on a blood test, and symptoms of a deficiency tend to be quite non-specific, but some people complain of tiredness, aches and pains. I will cover vitamin D in more detail in its own chapter.

There are lots of supplements on the market which are suitable for vegans. Many can be bought from the supermarket, but health food stores often supply more than one type. Calcium supplements are a bit contentious with the medical profession because associations have been made between hardening of arteries and calcium supplementation. So, as with many other micronutrients, obtaining your calcium from dietaty sources is always best.

On a final note, if your doctor has diagnosed you with thinning bones (osteopenia or osteoporosis), and is prescribing a vitamin D and calcium preparation, I am happy to tell you that there are two tablets which do not contain animal products. These are Calcichew D3 and Calcichew D3 forte, and your GP may be able to prescribe them for you, if appropriate.

10

Zinc

What is it and why do I need it?

Zinc isn't a mineral I usually include in my summaries for vegan health, or in my chats with patients. This is because it is readily available in many vegan-friendly foods, and isn't routinely tested for in day-to-day General Practice. However, there is some evidence that the zinc found in plant foods might not be as bioavailable as that in animal-derived sources, and that vegans could be at risk of deficiency.[349]

Zinc is a mineral which is involved in many bodily processes, including immune responses, cell turnover and growth, healing, and the absorption of other nutrients such as carbohydrates, fat and protein.

What's 'normal'?

From my own experience of working in General Practice, we don't often measure zinc levels, as most diets contain an abundance of it. However, it might be tested when there are other symptoms of, or conditions related to, malabsorption going on. It would usually be tested when somebody is under the care of a hospital team. A normal range for blood zinc levels is somewhere around 11–19 umol/l, and the recommended daily intake is between 5.5mg and 9.5mg for men, and 4mg and 7mg for women. Zinc is a micronutrient which can be harmful in overdose, so high dose supplements are not recommended.

What happens if I don't have enough?

Zinc deficiency is rare, and usually related to other nutritional deficiencies and diseases. But when it does occur, it comes with bowel disturbances, hair loss, altered taste and poor wound healing.

Where can vegans find it?

Zinc is found in many plant-based foods, but is in the highest quantities in lentils, tofu, chickpeas and beans, cashews and walnuts, and seeds including hemp, chia and linseeds. Some supplements targeted at vegans do, however, contain a dose of zinc, such as the one from The Vegan Society.

11

Iodine

What is it and why do I need it?

Iodine is an element which is essential in our bodies for the production of thyroid hormone. This is produced by the thyroid, a small gland which sits in the front of the neck, just above the notch in the top of the breast bone. Thyroid hormone regulates metabolism; this is the rate at which cells break down energy. Thyroid hormone also functions in babies and children for normal growth and mental development.

What's 'normal'?

It's quite difficult to measure iodine, and as such it's not done routinely or regularly in General Practice. But because iodine is excreted by the kidneys, levels can be checked by specialists, when necessary, by measuring the amount in urine.

Ordinarily, however, iodine status is checked by monitoring thyroid hormone levels. This is a blood test, and just to make things even more complicated, we don't necessarily use the level of thyroid hormone itself, but instead that of a hormone produced by the pituitary gland, called thyroid stimulating hormone, or TSH. When the thyroid is underactive, TSH levels go up, and when it is overactive, TSH levels go down. And just to complicate matters even more, many people with an iodine deficiency have an entirely normal thyroid function.

Current recommendations for iodine intake are 150mcg for adults, and 250mcg for those who are pregnant or breast(/chest) feeding.

What happens if I don't have enough?

Iodine deficiency leads to hypothyroidism – an underactive thyroid. This usually presents with tiredness, weight gain, dry skin and brittle hair, mental slowness and intolerance of the cold. It can also present with a goitre – a swelling of the thyroid gland which can be seen over the lower neck. The condition of hypothyroidism can also affect other bodily systems, for example leading to erectile dysfunction, heavy periods, constipation or a hoarse voice.

If a pregnancy occurs in an iodine-deficient person, congenital hypothyroidism, also known as Cretinism, can occur. This is, unfortunately, a serious condition which can result in growth problems and severe learning disabilities. It is tested for in the first days of life, however, and if present, rapid replacement of thyroid hormone can lead to normal intellectual development.

Where can vegans find it?

Iodine is usually sourced from seafood, meat and dairy products. It can be found in some vegetables; however, because the levels of iodine in soils can vary so much depending on location, they are difficult to predict from region to region. The best vegan source of iodine is sea vegetables, like seaweed. However, again, the actual content is very unpredictable, with levels of iodine in kelp varying from 16mcg to 165mcg per gram.

The safest way for vegans to get the right amount of iodine is by using fortified foods and supplementing. Safe, plant-based sources of iodine include fortified products like vegan milk and butter, but as many products are not fortified, the only truly safe way for us to ensure there is enough iodine in our diet is with supplements.

12

Vitamin B12 and Folate

What is it and why do I need it?

Both B12 and folate are in the group of B vitamins. The reason I bunch them together here, which might seem odd when folate deficiency is most definitely not a 'vegan' problem, is because they work closely together, and are often seen in deficiency together.

Vitamin B12, also called cobalamin, is used primarily in the production of red blood cells, but also in the process of wrapping nerves with myelin, the protective sheath that allows them to work efficiently. Folate is also known as vitamin B9, and it is also used in the process of blood cell production.

Both B12 and folate, when deficient, cause a type of anaemia which is classified as 'macrocytic', meaning that the blood cells increase in size to compensate. Macrocytosis isn't necessarily harmful in itself, but it does give clinicians a clue as to what the underlying cause of anaemia might be.

What's 'normal'?

B12 and folate levels are checked quite routinely with a blood test. A 'normal' B12 level can vary depending on the laboratory testing and reporting it, but generally it is anywhere from around 180 to 1000pg/ml. A mildly low B12 level might not be acted upon, but merely repeated after a short measure of time, perhaps 6 months.

The daily recommended dose of vitamin B12 is 1–2ug per day, but you will likely notice when shopping for supplements, that they contain much higher amounts, as it isn't very well absorbed. B12 is harmless in overdose, and readily excreted. Once deficient, however, a doctor will likely arrange a further test to ensure you don't have another condition called pernicious anaemia. This renders you unable to effectively absorb vitamin B12, and in cases of this, B12 injections will be prescribed instead.

Normal folate levels are usually over 4ng/ml, and daily requirements are 200mcg for both men and women.

What happens if I don't have enough?

The symptoms of either (or both) folate or B12 deficiency cause the same group of symptoms, because they both result in macrocytic anaemia. The most typical symptom is something called peripheral neuropathy: loss of feeling, tingling, numbness or pain in the peripheries, usually the feet. Other symptoms include fatigue, a sore, red tongue or redness at the corners of the mouth and ulcers in the mouth. There can also be psychological problems like depression, dementia and other cognitive disorders, and an eye condition called optic neuritis, which causes eye pain with loss of vision.

Where can vegans find it?

Whilst B12 is found in animal-derived foods, like meat, fish, dairy and eggs, folate is found mostly in plant foods like leafy, green vegetables, peas, beans and broccoli. Although B12 doesn't naturally occur in plant foods, many are fortified with it, such as plant milks, yeast extract and 'nooch', more properly known as nutritional yeast.

Because of the reduced exposure to B12 that vegans have, it is recommended that a regular supplement should be taken, unless you can be absolutely certain you obtain enough in your diet from fortified foods. Interestingly, B12 doesn't need to be taken every day, and can be consumed as a larger dose each week, or every few days.

Folate isn't usually on my list of recommended supplements for vegans, purely because it is so readily available in a healthy vegan diet. An exception to this is pregnant people who must take folic acid supplements for the first 3 months of pregnancy to prevent spina bifida associated with folate deficiency, hopefully having been counselled to take it pre-conception.

13

Vitamin D

What is it and why do I need it?

Vitamin D, also called calciferol, or the sunshine vitamin for reasons I'll explain below, is a fat-soluble vitamin, which means that it is found within fatty foods and is much better absorbed when consumed with dietary fats. Vitamin D helps the absorption of calcium in the gut, as well as regulating blood calcium levels, so it is really important for bone health. Vitamin D is also involved in many processes throughout the body including reducing inflammation, the immune system, and cell growth and division.

What's 'normal'?

Vitamin D levels are measured frequently by GPs in the UK, particularly because deficiency is very common, primarily due to us living in a climate that isn't very sunny. Levels should be more than 50 nmol/L, and anything less than this can be divided into either insufficiency or deficiency.

Vitamin D deficiency is diagnosed when levels go below 25nmol/L, but anything between 25 and 49nmol/L is classified as an insufficiency, whilst a level of 50nmol/L or above is required for good health. Vitamin D is one of the vitamins which can be overdosed on, and although this is quite rare, a measurement of more than 125nmol/L can be dangerous, as it is associated with raised calcium levels, which can be very serious, and even fatal.

What happens if I don't have enough?

Vitamin D deficiency is more common in some groups of people, including those over 65 years old or who are housebound, people with darker skin pigmentation, anyone having undergone weight loss surgery, and pregnant and breast(/chest) feeding people. You can also become deficient if you cover up your skin, reducing your exposure to sunlight.

Deficiency of vitamin D can often be asymptomatic, and only found when blood levels have been tested for other reasons. But some people can experience widespread aches and pains, muscle weakness, and localised bone pains.

If it is left untreated, vitamin D deficiency can lead to osteomalacia in adults, and rickets in children. Both of these conditions involve the loss of bone mass, leading to fractures and bone deformities.

Where can vegans find it?

Vitamin D is found in some foods, but is also made in our skin when it is exposed to sunlight. And this is why it is known as the sunshine vitamin. Short periods of time in the sun with arms and shoulders exposed should be enough to get your daily dose of vitamin D, but darker skinned people may need a little longer. It's really important not to spend prolonged periods of time in the sun without protection, like SPF and a hat though, as too much sun exposure can also lead to skin cancers.

But if you live in a rainy country, where we can't always rely on the sun being around, or if you are unable to get out into it, you might need to look at dietary sources and supplements. It is important to note, however, that most sources aren't vegan. However, there are fortified foods, like plant milks, which have it added.

Because of the poor dietary availability of vitamin D in vegan foods, and the unreliability of the British weather, I recommend all vegans take a supplement. There are specifically vegan multivitamins which contain it, along with other vegan essentials, or you can buy it on its own, or combined with calcium. The issue with taking a supplement, however, is that unless it specifies a vegan source, it is usually made from lanolin from sheep's wool. Please be reassured, though, there are many vegan options on the market, you just need to check.

14

All the Rest

(Well, some of them, anyway.)

There are so many micronutrients, that it would be difficult to cover all of them in this book. But, to be honest, we don't need to. I've covered everything that you might miss with a vegan diet, but as you can probably tell by now, balance and planning is the key. This chapter is just to include a few of the other commonly considered micronutrients, those which we can become deficient in, but not because of a vegan diet. If I've not mentioned a particular micronutrient, it's because deficiency is either unlikely or unheard of, whether in vegans, or more generally.

If you're physically well and eating with care, I wouldn't give the rest of these mentioned micronutrients too much thought.

Minerals

Magnesium

Like calcium, magnesium is an element which is also essential for healthy bones and soft tissues, and is similarly used by the nervous system in relaying nerve impulses. It is abundant in a balanced diet, being found in most foods that contain fibre, and being added to some fortified foods, like breakfast cereals. Low magnesium isn't that uncommon, and can occur with lots of medical conditions. It can be tested for by your GP and replaced, if necessary.

Potassium

Potassium is another element used in lots of cellular functions within the body. There are no real concerns about deficiency, because again, it is found in abundance in most diets. In a vegan diet we would find potassium in bananas, dried fruits, coffee, tomatoes, mushrooms, sweetcorn and many other vegetables, chocolate, nuts and crisps. Certain medical conditions and medications can cause a low level, however, and this is called hypokalaemia. In this instance, a doctor may prescribe a potassium replacement.

Selenium

This is an antioxidant mineral, which is used by enzymes for several processes within the body. Vegans can find it in grains, mushrooms, Brazil nuts and garlic. Selenium deficiency only occurs in two specific situations:[350] where deficiency is endemic, for example in a very specific area of China, and in patients who rely on TPN (total parenteral nutrition), where all nutrition is given to a person intravenously) who aren't also given selenium supplementation. I've never tested for selenium deficiency, nor have I treated it.

Sodium

Sodium, found in many, many foods and in table salt as sodium chloride, is a mineral used in water balance throughout the body. Deficiency doesn't really occur, and actually we need to be rather careful not to consume too much. But we often do find low levels on a blood test, known as hyponatraemia. But this isn't dietary, nor really a deficiency, and would be related to electrolyte balance because of kidney function. I mention it here as an aside, because you may have heard of low sodium levels.

Vitamins

Vitamin A

Vitamin A is an antioxidant, meaning it can be protective against cardiovascular disease and cancer. It is a fat soluble vitamin, found in many foods, and interestingly, while those in the global north obtain theirs from animal-derived foods, the rest of the world gets their vitamin A from plant sources like oranges, carrots, and yellow peppers, where it is contained as beta-carotene.[351] We don't often see deficiency of vitamin A, and I've never seen it tested for or treated. However, an important note to make is that it is dangerous in excess in pregnant women, and supplements should be avoided.

Vitamin B1

This water-soluble vitamin is also known as thiamine. It is found in many foods, but for vegans these are primarily grains, nuts and yeast. Because it is found everywhere, thiamine deficiency is usually from starvation, or in alcohol-dependent people who aren't eating well. So

I do often prescribe it for my patients, but not for those who are well and eating a balanced diet.

Vitamin B2

Also known as riboflavin, B2 is in the group of B vitamins which act as co-enzymes in lots of processes throughout the body. It is found in legumes and pulses, and deficiency is only usually seen in starvation or alcohol dependence. There's no simple blood test for it, and it isn't a deficiency we usually investigate for.

Vitamin B6

Vitamin B6, also called pyridoxine, is also a co-enzyme, found in whole grains, yeast, tomato, corn and spinach. This is another vitamin for which deficiency is rather rare, and would be related to medical conditions rather than dietary intake.

Vitamin C

Another water-soluble vitamin, vitamin C has many roles, but most importantly for vegans, is its role in the absorption of iron. It is found in many vegan foods, including citrus fruits, tomatoes and green vegetables. Vitamin C is another antioxidant vitamin, meaning it might protect from cardiovascular disease and cancer. Deficiency causes scurvy, a condition which is now, thankfully, extremely rare, and related to lack of intake of fresh fruits and vegetables. I mention vitamin C intake more because of its relevance to vegans in helping us to absorb iron.

Vitamin E

Another antioxidant, but this time fat-soluble, vitamin E is important for muscle development and in reproductive processes. This is found primarily in plant foods and good sources include fresh nuts and green leafy vegetables. Vitamin E deficiency is rare in humans, but excessive supplementation has been associated with all-cause mortality.[352]

Vitamin K

Vitamin K is a group of fat-soluble vitamins, including K1 and K2. The main role of these is in blood clotting. Vegan sources are abundant, and include leafy vegetables, some legumes and rapeseed oil. Deficiency isn't usually seen because of dietary reasons, other than in starvation. When it does occur it causes bleeding.

GETTING STARTED

15

What Should I Do First?

So now you've read through the first four chapters, and you've learned all about how veganism is the better choice for animal welfare, for climate change, for human health, and for the rights of marginalised people, you've got no choice but to become vegan, right? But where do you start? It seems like a mammoth task, doesn't it? But it's very possible.

The internet's plant-based forums are full of very zealous vegans who berate people for congratulating others on their 'journey' to veganism. Many believe that for every day that you're just contemplating change, or working towards veganism, it is unreasonable that animals are still being farmed and slaughtered for your dietary choices. Whilst I absolutely believe that this has to change, and that every farmed animal should be free, and that we should be making more compassionate choices for ourselves and the planet, I also think that these changes should be sustainable. That you should be able to maintain your veganism, to understand how you are going to do it, and that you should be comfortable enough to be able to keep doing it.

So don't try to change everything overnight if this is too frightening. Start by cutting out meat, for example. Then a couple of weeks later once you are comfy with the vegetarian choices you are making, cut out dairy. Or vice versa. Then eggs can go. Or concentrate on your diet, cut all of the animal products out there, then look at your household items.

'What?! I need to change all of my household items, too?' I hear you ask. Well, remember I said that veganism is a lifestyle, not a diet? Your cleaning and beauty products are examples of items that need also need to be ensured to be cruelty-free, not containing animal products, and just generally not reliant on the exploitation of animals in order to be produced. But don't worry, this can come next, and there is a chapter a little later to help you with this.

Start by having a look at the 'Shopping Lists and Store Cupboard Staples' a little later in this section, and you might be surprised with the amount of vegan-friendly items already lurking in your cupboards. If you're comfortable to do so after reading the information I've presented you with, then use up the non-vegan items you have, and make sure the next lot you buy are vegan-friendly. If you don't like the idea of using those chicken thighs from the fridge now you understand the pain and suffering that was involved in their production, then donate them to somebody else who would eat them. If your friends and family don't want them, pop them on a Facebook free-items page, or in an app like Olio. Although I'm long past eating anything that's come from an animal, I hate the idea of waste, especially when somebody has died for that item.

Another good thing to do is to tell people around you, especially any vegans you know. It's good to get the support of others, and it's great for accountability. Of course you will need to let people know so that when you spend time together they will be aware that you won't be able to eat anything non-vegan. And, of course you're going to be accused of telling everybody that you're vegan. It's par for the course. But don't worry, just laugh it off. If you don't tell people, they'd give you non-vegan foods to eat, and if you do tell people you get laughed at for always talking about veganism. That's just going to become a fact of life now.

Once you've made the transition and your fridge is full of vegan food, and you're happy that you are going to be cooking just plant-based meals from now on, make sure that you've got your supplements ready to start taking. You will probably have read the nutrition chapters by now, but just to recap, I recommend that all vegans take:

- Vitamin B12
- Vitamin D
- Iodine
- Omega-3 — preferably DHA and EPA

You can take these separately, or you can buy a supplement with all of the vitamins and minerals in. Omegas never come combined with these, so you will have to supplement this separately. For the vitamins and minerals, I like to take the one from The Vegan Society, but I also quite like some of the sprays you can buy. Omega-3s often come in a chewable gummy, or a drop you put into your food or drink.

Then it's time to start exploring vegan products. Milk is a good place to begin, as it is often a staple in most people's fridges. There is a lot of variation between the different plant milks, and some will suit different uses better than others. For example, the barista style oat milks work well in coffees, and I really liked them for my children when they were moving away from breast milk, as they have a higher fat content than other plant milks, and are fortified with calcium, iodine and vitamin D. But I much prefer soya milk in a cup of tea, and I like the health benefits of soya, so if I need to use a large volume of milk to make a sauce or pancakes, for example, then I'll put soya milk in there.

Now, I say this with all seriousness: don't switch over to vegan cheese until you're mentally ready. The cheese situation is a lot better than when I went vegan back in 2017. But if you get it wrong on your first try, you might scar yourself for life. You're much better having a period of abstinence, learning all about veganism and nailing the other aspects of your diet, then coming back to cheese once you well and truly feel like a vegan. If, like me, you were a cheese hound before transitioning, choose wisely. Spend some money on an artisan vegan cheese; there are some brilliant, albeit a bit expensive, dairy-free cheeses, and these are usually made from cashews, and they are often fermented and cultured in the same way as dairy cheese. For your first try, it really is worth splashing out where you can. Once your palate has adjusted, just go explore. Most of the soft cheeses are very easy to eat and use, and there are widely available cheddar-style hard cheeses made from coconut, which are great for a sandwich or salad. Exploring all of these new products can really be exciting and fun. It's a whole new world of food.

Do you remember the wellbeing section in the 'Vegan for Health' chapter, and how we discussed that a sense of belonging can improve your your health? Well, in order to really harness this, you need to seek out your tribe. You can find fellow vegans on various social media platforms, and depending on what will suit you more, you can either follow vegan influencers for guidance, advice and motivation, or you can join groups so you can ask questions, chat, and generally feel part of a group. There's also lots of great books on veganism, which can help you to keep going, offer inspiration for cooking, and advise you how to argue with meat eaters. I'll include as many of these as I can in the 'Useful Resources' chapter.

16

So, Do I Need to See My Doctor?

We've already had a look at all the deficiencies we might encounter if we're not careful with our vegan diet. But we've also read about just how healthy a plant-based diet can be. So if you're switching from an omnivorous diet to a vegan one, do you need to see your doctor?

The answer is probably not. If you're taking a well-balanced vegan diet, and supplementing with the essentials, like vitamins B12 and D, iodine and omega-3, then you're probably going to be just fine, nutritionally speaking. I think perhaps the only exception to this is if you're diabetic and on blood-sugar lowering medications, then I would considering chatting to your diabetes nurse, GP, or specialist first, as your new diet might be so healthful and your calorie intake so different, that you could be at risk of hypoglycaemia, or low blood sugars. You might even need to see your healthcare professional to have your medication lowered or stopped!

Otherwise I would suggest that you see your GP if you've been on your vegan diet for some time, and you experience any symptoms of deficiency, which are, broadly, tiredness, headaches, hair thinning, nail changes, a sore mouth or lips, shortness of breath, chest pain on exertion, and tingling of the limbs. But, as I've mentioned previously, I would hope that anyone experiencing these symptoms for any significant length of time would see their GP for an examination and some investigations whether they had been living on a vegan diet or not. If anything doesn't feel quite right, it's fine to speak to your GP, mention that you are vegan, and suggest that you might like to have some blood tests done to check for potential deficiencies.

So that brings me on to my next point. How to talk to your GP, or any healthcare professional, about being vegan. It makes me really sad when I hear vegans tell me that they've been too frightened to tell their healthcare provider that they follow a vegan lifestyle. Many vegans are very compassionate, thoughtful and reflective individuals. Most vegans have pure intention behind their decision to follow the lifestyle, whether that is for the animals, or to help save our wonderful planet. Apart from the fact that I think all patients should be listened to, treated with respect, and leave a doctor's room feeling heard and understood, nobody should be met with disdain or be laughed at for their philosophies and beliefs.

I've often thought that vegans ought to earn some kind of respect from our peers and neighbours on this planet for our decision to live this way. We're doing what everybody needs to be doing in order for the planet to survive, and for animals to finally get the rights that they deserve. But unfortunately, the world doesn't yet see it this way. I've heard people saying that when you tell somebody you are vegan, it is like holding up a mirror to their behaviours and lifestyle. This is why we're often ridiculed. Because ridicule and projecting your annoyance is easier than questioning how you live, and whether it is time to make significant changes towards improving this planet for everybody. And doctors are no different. They are merely a snapshot of the rest of society. Some will be enthusiastic carnivores, believing the latest trends about the carnivore and keto diets. I do find this disappointing, to be honest, because the scientific evidence is there for everybody to see if they just learn how to critically appraise a paper. Many doctors, however, won't pay too much attention to how they live and what they eat, much like the majority of society. And a few will be vegan, understanding all the implications, complications and benefits.

If you are unfortunate enough to meet with a healthcare professional who doesn't understand what being a vegan means, or worse still, believes that it is unhealthy or unsafe, what can you do?

Firstly, you need to remind any professional who is discriminatory against your choice to follow a vegan lifestyle that it is a protected characteristic.[353] If you have a really unpleasant experience, you can ask to see a different health professional next time, if there is another one available in that particular field of expertise. Then it might be a good idea to clear up what veganism means; sometimes people just don't understand, and a quick explanation about what it is, and why you've chosen this way of life might just be enough to get your consultation back on track. The final thing you can do, which could make your life easier, but also has the potential to change the life of not just the professional sitting in front of you, but every patient that comes after you, is to point them towards the evidence. I'll put lots of information and links for the various helpful websites in the 'Useful Resources' chapter at the end of the book, but here is a quick list that your health professionals might find helpful. At the very least, they won't be easily able to scoff at your choices, once they've seen what these experts have got to say about plant-based eating and veganism:

- The Vegan Doctor
- Plant-Based Health Professionals UK
- Physicians Committee for Responsible Medicine
- Dr Michael Greger of Nutrition Facts

- EAT-Lancet Report
- The Vegan Society

And with this sharing of information, your activism journey begins.

17

Debunking Those Vegan Myths

Veganism isn't safe for children and babies.

I could just give you anecdotal evidence from all the vegan children and babies I've treated and known, including my own, but I'll provide you with something a little more formalised and concrete: the British Dietetic Association states that a plant-based diet can support healthy living at every age and life stage.[354]

You can't get enough protein on a vegan diet.

Hopefully you've read the section on nutrition by now. If not, go back and take a look. I think it will reassure you that there is plenty of protein in plants, and some contain more than others. So if you're particularly concerned, then turn to the high protein foods like beans, tofu, lentils and peas. And if you are body-building, and really requiring a very high protein intake, there are plenty of vegan protein powders on the market, but most people really don't need to use these.

You need to eat dairy for calcium.

Again, please take a look at the chapter on calcium, where you will find lots of information about calcium-rich plant foods, and learn that you definitely don't need dairy for this. Not only do plant sources of calcium avoid the saturated fat of many dairy ones, but you can also avoid the potential of increased risk of certain cancers and improve your bone health by avoiding dairy.

Plant-based iron isn't adequate.

The iron chapter of this book tells us all about how non-haem iron is slightly harder for the human body to absorb than animal-derived haem iron, but there are also tips on how to improve its absorption, and how to find a wealth of iron in a plant-based diet. My chapter on 'Vegan for Health' will also help you to understand that haem iron from animals comes with several health risks, so iron from plants is preferable, and most definitely adequate.

You can't go cold turkey from meat and dairy.

I'm not sure the use of the phrase 'cold turkey' is appropriate when talking about veganism! But again, this is a myth. You absolutely can jump straight into veganism. Some people might find this easier, and some people who aren't used to taking a lot of fibre in their diet might find that their bowels take a while to get used to eating much more. If this is the case, slow down on the fibre, and don't forget what I've said about cheese! I would definitely go cold turkey on the cheese for a while, then introduce that once you're happy to try vegan versions.

Pregnant people can't be vegan.

I'm going to direct you back to the statement from the BDA again for this one, as it confirms that veganism is suitable for *every* life stage. From a personal perspective, I have done two healthy pregnancies whilst vegan, which were difficult at times, but perfectly manageable, with a healthy baby born at the end of both.

Veganism is expensive.

This one is slightly trickier to debunk, as veganism can be expensive. But it doesn't have to be. Some of the vegan meat replacements are expensive, but honestly, they are comparable to meat. Unless you are buying very cheap meat, and the health effects of this and its impact on animal welfare and the planet is very questionable, so I certainly wouldn't be comparing your plant-based foods to this. As I hope you're starting to understand, the healthiest way of eating is a whole-food plant-based diet, and this is possible to do very cheaply. You can use dried foods like beans, soya mince and lentils which can be used in many dishes, and you can buy big bags of these from most supermarkets. However, fresh fruits, nuts and seeds are where you'll easily spend a lot of money, as these aren't cheap. But these items aren't exclusive to a vegan diet, and should be consumed by everybody. Honestly, eating good quality food is expensive, generally, in the current economic climate. But eating vegan should be no more expensive than eating omnivorously, and could be done cheaper with bulk-bought, batch-cooked whole foods.

Vegan food is all ultra-processed.

The answer to this is going to be similar to the myth above. Vegan food is as ultra-processed as omnivorous food. Yes, you could be vegan and eat only ultra-processed foods, but equally you can be omnivorous or vegetarian and eat only ultra-processed too. Once again, I'm going to suggest that you aim to head towards a target of being as close to whole-food plant-based as possible, and this is where true health and wellbeing lies.

Vegans don't need to take any supplements.

No matter how healthy and close to WFPB your diet is, there are some nutrients that aren't as available in a vegan diet, so to be sure you're not at risk of deficiency, supplements should be taken. I've mentioned which ones to concentrate on before, but I'll pop them here again:

- Vitamin B12
- Vitamin D
- Iodine
- Omega-3 (DHA)

Of course you need to tailor your diet and supplements to your personal needs, and there are other nutrients that you need to think about in your day-to-day food intake, but these are the four that I would seriously consider taking as a daily supplement.

I can't take medications because they aren't vegan.

Even if medications don't contain animal-derived ingredients, none of them can be called vegan, because all medication in the UK needs to be tested on animals, by law. Sadly there is no way around this, and it doesn't appear to be changing any time soon. But it's important to remember that most vegans consider medication to be exempt from the philosophy of veganism, because by The Vegan Society's definition, veganism is only 'as far as is possible and practicable'. And if medications have to be tested on animals to be licensed in the UK, then we don't have any control over the fact that they aren't vegan. I would argue it is important to take essential medications to maintain health and be able to continue your good work and positive messages of veganism. Please see the medication section of the 'What About Non-Food Items' chapter, for more information on managing medications as a vegan.

Vegan diets are always healthy.

In the same way that it is a complete myth that vegan diets are full of ultra-processed foods, they aren't always healthy either. It is possible for a vegan diet to be both or neither of these things. Most vegans have a diet somewhere in the middle, which is a good place to aim for as a starting point, but incorporating as many whole foods as possible into your diet is preferable. Whilst all vegan diets are not healthy, and the odd treat of junk foods or treats is OK, I would be aiming for a truly plant-rich diet.

Vegan diets are harmful to the environment

This book has touched on the environment, and the impact of meat and dairy upon it. However, vegans often hear the argument (usually from staunch carnivores) that veganism is harmful to the environment. I won't repeat everything I've told you already, but just to recap: plants, including soya, use far less land and water than meat production, and produce fewer carbon emissions. Soya is often given as a reason why vegan diets are worse for the earth. But, as I told you previously, most soya is fed to farmed animals that are destined for the dinner plates of meat-eaters. Almonds and avocados also come under fire, and, like soya, it's an interesting choice to point fingers at vegans, because I'm sure most of the people I know who eat both of these foods regularly, aren't vegan. I quite like the summary given by Viva! about why avocados aren't as harmful as some would have you believe:[355]

- Avocados grow on trees, which capture CO_2.
- A single avocado requires 140–272 litres of water. The same amount of beef requires 2,315 litres of water.
- Avocados are transported by sea, which has a smaller carbon footprint than air travel – 'Even when shipped at great distances, its [avocado's] emissions are much less than locally-produced animal products.'

The reason why almonds have been singled out as being so bad for the earth is because of their very high water requirements. Again, it's not just vegans who eat almonds, but almond milk is often used as an alternative to dairy (by vegans and non-vegans, alike), so this is probably why those of us who eat plant-based are accused of consuming earth-harmful foods. But, when compared to dairy, the water requirements of almond milk, litre for litre, is 10 times less.[356] The bottom line is that a vegan diet is, in no way, worse for the environment than an omnivorous one.

Humans are supposed to eat meat

This argument is often thrown about with very little evidence, or worse still, whilst the person providing it is pointing at their almost non-existent canines. I'm not sure what qualifies most people to argue that we're supposed to eat meat. If it were true, why would the more essential nutrients that we require only be found in plants, like fibre, vitamin C, and antioxidants? The only nutrient we can't get from plants is B12, but even this is often only found in meat because of supplementation of farmed animals. Humans are meant to be omnivorous, meaning we can eat animals or plants. But when we live in a modern society where all nutrition is available to us without the mass slaughter and cruel factory farming involved in meat production, why would you choose to consume anything but plants?

18

Plant-Based Pitfalls

It's inevitable: you will be congratulating yourself on nailing this veganism lark, and then someone will point out – maybe even gleefully – that your sandwich bread contains milk… I think the main thing here is not to worry too much about falling into traps as you set out on your journey to becoming vegan. As long as you're not allergic to any ingredients, you might have to just accept that accidental slip-ups will happen, at least at the start. It doesn't make you any less vegan, and your intentions are still good. But to keep them to a minimum, let's look at what some of those traps are.

Milk/dairy

It's a standing joke among vegans that everything, and I mean everything, contains milk. In reality, it's not a joke. It's really frustrating. And when you first start out, you'll probably get caught out so many times. One thing that works in vegans' favour, fortunately, is that because milk is an allergen, every version of it is listed and usually highlighted on an ingredient list. You might see it called, simply, milk. Alternatively, you might see lactose on the list, but anything milk-related should always be highlighted as an allergen.

Egg

This one is often lurking in gluten-free breads, and I have been caught out several times. Again, it is an allergen, so it is always highlighted when present. Also be cautious of egg-containing pastas and noodles; it's usually fresh pasta that contains egg, and, rather sensibly, egg-containing noodles are often called 'egg noodles'. But I would suggest you still check the ingredient list before buying.

Gelatine

This is a substance made from rendered down collagen-containing connective tissues from animals. Yes, it is as disgusting as it sounds. It's made from hair, hooves and tendons. As the name suggests, it makes a gelatinous substance, so it is used in things that are chewy or set, like sweets and puddings. Just check your chewy sweets and traditional desserts like panna cotta.

Additives

You will have seen those E numbers on your ingredient lists, and you may try to avoid them, believing that they are all chemical additives. Well many of them are, but some are also derived from animals, or even insects. The ones to watch out for are:

- E120 – this is cochineal, a red colouring made from ground up beetles
- E542 – bone phosphate, made from crushed bone
- E901 – beeswax
- E904 – shellac, made from beetles (not the same as the nail care brand)
- E913 – lanolin, made from sheep's wool

- E966 – lactitol, a sweetener made from milk
- E1105 – lysozyme, an enzyme from egg whites

'Plant-based'

This is a confusing one, and it caught me out once. Sometimes restaurants and pubs list something like a burger as 'plant-based', when it isn't necessarily vegan. For example, it may be made with a technically vegan patty, but the mayo and cheese on it might be made from milk and egg. One way around this is to ask the kitchen to leave the non-vegan item off. Another issue is that some restaurants will cook what would have been a vegan item in the same oil or on the same grill as non-vegan items. I think whether you want to eat this is a really personal decision. For me, I am no less vegan because I eat an item that was next to meat. I have still avoided the items that have come from a place of pain and suffering, and my choice is still better for me and the planet.

Honey

Honey is a popular foodstuff, often touted as having health-promoting properties, and being a natural alternative to refined sugar. Apart from the risk to young babies, who can catch botulism from consuming honey, I don't know of any other negative health implications for it. The reason vegans exclude it, however, is that it's harvested from bees through exploitative and cruel methods. I think honey and beekeeping has a rather romantic image, but the reality is very different from this. Honey is made by bees from the nectar they collect from flowers, and is their main nutrient source. It is stored for use later on, but beekeepers remove it, replacing the honey with sugar water, a far less nutritious alternative. This leaves the bees unhealthy and at risk of disease. The keeping of bees is also quite unnatural, and requires manipulation of their natural lives. Methods to remove honey from the hive can result in harm and even death to members of the hive, and it's not uncommon for beekeepers to cull their hive in the winter to save money. Queen bees are on the end of nasty practices like artificial insemination and wing clipping in order to allow a hive to produce honey. There are implications for the wider natural world too, however. Not unlike farmed mammals, bees are bred for productivity, meaning that there is also a similar picture of reduced diversity, which can have far-reaching impacts on the environment, because bees have a very important role in pollination.

Some people who follow a vegan lifestyle choose to continue consuming honey, often at the criticism of other vegans. When I know how the practices involved in honey harvesting harm the bees and our natural world, I choose not to include it in my diet. I also avoid it in other products, like cosmetics and medicines, which is where many vegans might get tripped up.

Quorn Products

Whilst some Quorn products are brilliant, and can be a great source of protein, not all of their products are actually vegan-friendly. Many are just vegetarian and contain egg, much to the frustration of many vegans. Annoyingly, they have even changed some of their vegan products back to being just vegetarian! So, if you're choosing Quorn products, just be careful to check the ingredients list if it doesn't specify on the front of the pack that it's a vegan product.

19

Store Cupboard Staples

Sometimes it's hard to get started on a new way of doing any-thing, let alone eating. It's something we do, literally, to survive, and several times a day. So making adjustments to this can be daunt-ing. To help you get started, here's a list of ingredients which you will find useful to have in your pantry, either because they are in lots of recipes, or because you'll gain a lot from eating them regularly.

Agave syrup

Whilst syrups are, in no way, an essential food, since I've been vegan, I've found that many recipes call for honey as a natural sweetener, and agave is a very good substitute. Other syrups are great for sweet-ening food without using refined sugar include maple and date syrups.

Beans

I almost feel like I shouldn't be allowed to call beans 'beans', in one short word, like they're all just the same thing. The variety of beans is so vast, that there is a whole universe of these delicious little pack-ages of goodness to discover. When I'm giving nutrition advice to my patients now, I just tell them to put beans in everything. Well, I offer other insights, too, but I really can't exaggerate the benefits of beans. They are just fabulous for our health, and it is a bonus that they are so tasty, too. Personal favourites of mine include haricot, borlotti and butter beans. But, seriously, go wild, try them all.

Cashews

Although cashews are often found in bags of mixed nuts, every vegan should have a bag of raw cashews in their pantry. They can be soaked and blended to make cheese, white sauces, or just to add a creamy element to any dish. Not to mention that they are delicious in a curry!

Chia seeds

Chia seeds have a great function in cooking and baking, being an alternative to flaxseeds as an egg replacement, but they are also a good source of fibre, protein, omega-3 fatty acids, and antioxidants. I also quite like the crunch unsoaked chia add to some dishes!

Chickpeas

No vegan food cupboard should be without a can of chickpeas. They are a very versatile source of protein and fibre, that can be thrown into or onto pretty much any meal. And don't forget that you can stick them in a blender with a splash of oil and some tahini for a delicious, fresh houmous (see my recipe on page 255). And you may not know this, but the liquid that chickpeas come in, called aquafaba, can be whipped up into a meringue, mayonaise, or used in a chocolate mousse in place of egg whites. Just make sure that you haven't picked up chickpeas in salted water.

Dark chocolate

I think every treat cupboard should contain a good quality dark chocolate, vegan household or not. Many of us like to finish a meal with something sweet, and whilst fruit is just perfect, there's something about chocolate, isn't there? But dark chocolate is actually really, really good for you. Make it a high cocoa percentage, and low sugar, and your body will thank you for the beautiful antioxidants the chocolate contains, and your tastebuds will thank you for the decadent hit of sweetness. There really is no need to miss out on favourites because you've gone vegan.

Extra virgin olive oil

This isn't really a vegan rule, but one for everybody. Good quality extra virgin olive oil is known for its healthful qualities, and is great for drizzling and making salad dressings. You can also cook with it for a healthier choice, but the olive flavour might be too powerful for some dishes that don't necessarily suit it. Many of the benefits of the Mediterranean Diet seen in the studies we discussed earlier are from the inclusion of extra virgin olive oil.

Flours

Plain flour and self-raising are great staples for so many different dishes, but important additions to the vegan cupboard are gram (chickpea) flour and cornflour. Gram flour can be used to make omelette-style dishes, and with a little kala namak from your spice cupboard, you've got a very tasty brunch. Cornflour is great for making the texture of tofu a bit more interesting; just rolling cubes of tofu in seasoned cornflour before frying them can really crisp them up a treat.

Grains

I've only really discovered the wonderful world of grains since I started eating more WFPB. Of course I knew something about rices, and I have loved pearl barley since childhood (importantly, this isn't a whole grain, because it has been polished so the outer layers have been removed), but I didn't yet know about bulgur wheat, buckwheat, quinoa and spelt. Of course there are plenty more, but I love these in particular, and I sometimes use them as a replacement where I previously would have had a potato or pasta side dish, or as the base for a great salad. Being wholegrain, they are full of wonderful health-promoting properties, as well as being delicious and satisfying.

Ground/milled flaxseed

Seeds really are getting a look-in in this section, aren't they? Milled flax (or linseed) are used in an similar way to chia seeds for binding foods, and as a great source of omega-3. It's so easy to boost your omega-3 intake with a spoonful of milled flaxseed in a soup or sauce. You'll notice in my recipe section, that flaxseed are my go-to egg replacement.

Herbs

I always buy a selection of fresh herbs with my shopping each week including mint, dill, thyme and coriander. They are essential for some of my recipes, but they are also delicious chopped into salads and sandwiches. Many dishes which have been 'veganised' rely on certain flavour profiles from herbs and spices, so there are a few pots of dried herbs that I always have in my cupboard:

- thyme
- rosemary
- sage
- parsley
- oregano

Lentils

The variety of lentils, as far as I'm aware, isn't quite on the same scale as beans, but there are a surprising number of types to try. Each has its own properties that it offers your meal, and so I tend to use each one differently. I like red lentils in soups, curries and blended into sauces, and I like green lentils as a minced meat substitute, thrown into salads and in casseroles. Puy lentils I have for a treat, because they are rich and peppery, and delicious as a side dish by themselves. If you're not sure about cooking them, start with tins or pouches of already prepared lentils. It's a great way to discover how you like to use them best.

Marmite

One of the flavours that can be lost when you're not cooking with animal products is 'umami' so finding a way of adding this back in with plant-based products is welcome. I think that marmite, or other brands of yeast extract, can add a wonderful depth of flavour. If you are worried about the salt content, low sodium versions are available.

Miso paste

I discovered delicious miso paste when I was making a Japanese broth. Once I had tasted it, I started putting it into other soups, sauces and dishes for an amazing umami hit. It's made from fermented soya beans, meaning it also has some health benefits, being great for your microbiome, and therefore having other knock-on effects for the rest of your health. I even enjoy it as a hot drink, sometimes (think of pre-vegan Bovril on a wintery night).

Mixed nuts

Whilst this isn't on the list for my recipes, it's here because nuts are an essential snack. They're full of fibre, protein, vitamins, minerals and a great source of healthy fats. Some people avoid them because of their high fat content, but evidence seems to show that they don't cause weight gain when eaten moderately as a healthy snack. I often recommend to my patients that they should replace salty, low nutritional value snacks with a handful of delicious nuts. Raw is preferable, but even roasted and salted is better than a bag of crisps for your health.

Mixed seeds

A bag of mixed seeds offer a crunchy, nutritious boost to salads, poke bowls and buddha bowls. They can contain a good dose of omega-3 fatty acids, protein and fibre, as well as other vitamins and minerals.

Noodles and pasta

It might seem surprising that I'm putting noodles pasta here, as I'm sure they are found in everybody's cupboard anyway. They are cheap, quick to cook, and popular with kids and adults, alike. They're also really versatile. But I include them here because I often hear the words 'oh, I've never tried vegan food', and I often want to reply with, 'so, you've never eaten pasta (or rice, or noodles, or bread, or apples, etc., etc., etc.)?' When starting out on your vegan journey, it's often easy to forget about some of the reliable foods that have been there for you forever. And that some of these are more nutritious than you might realise. Even plain old white pasta has fibre, protein, vitamins and minerals in it. You can increase the nutrient content by using brown pasta instead, or increase your protein intake by switching to a lentil-flour pasta. Just be sure to avoid the egg-containing fresh pastas. When buying noodles, also consider buying wholemeal versions, and again avoid egg noodles. For variety (and some of my recipes) do get yourself some lovely chewy udon noodles, a range of rice noodles, which come as thin vermicelli style, or larger flat noodles, and my absolute favourite, Korean glass noodles, which are made from sweet potato flour.

Nut butters

The good old familiar one is peanut butter, which has just so much versatility, adding flavour and healthy fat to so many dishes. But you can also buy almond butter very easily, and if you're near a health food shop, you might even find cashew and hazelnut butter, which all have great health benefits, and make a fab snack smeared onto toast or apple slices for you or your little one.

Nutritional yeast

Also lovingly nicknamed *nooch*, this is a product which is well-loved by vegans around the world. It comes in flakes, and looks a bit like fish food. But it's got a nutty, cheesy flavour, and works well added to all kinds of foods including cheese sauces, bolognese or soups. It's a great source of vitamin B12, the main reason why vegans use it in everything, but it also contains fibre, zinc and all of the other B vitamins.

Plant milk

There are now so many different plant milks on the market, from good old soya milk (sweetened and unsweetened), to oat milk, almond, coconut, and hazelnut. Each has its own qualities, whether it is a creamy, smooth texture for using in a puddings or pancakes, or a nutty flavour for making an autumnal latte. You might end up relying on one that you like in everything, or having a carton of one or two different varieties for different purposes. I know that there are few loose rules, though, that many vegans seem to agree on:

- Soya milk for a good cup of tea
- Barista style oat milk for coffee
- Barista milks for transitioning babies and toddlers off breast milk

Rapeseed oil

Rapeseed oil has a bit of a mixed reputation, mostly because there is a group of whole-food plant-based type vegans who avoid oil completely. There is one school of thought which states that vegetable and seed oils are inflammatory in nature, but the evidence for this doesn't really seem to stand up.[357] There's also the fact that oils are very calorie dense, meaning that consuming just small amounts provides a high amount of calories, but perhaps little other nutrition.

But most evidence shows that plant-based oils are safe, and definitely better than saturated fats like butter, tallow and lard.[358] A good quality rapeseed oil is a great source of omega-3, which as we've already learned in the nutrition section, is particularly important in a vegan diet. For the absolutely best quality, you should buy cold-pressed rapeseed oil, which is also great on salads and in dressings, but is expensive. But supermarkets' own vegetable oil is usually just rapeseed oil, and will also provide omega-3.

Rice

Rice is another staple for everyone, vegan or not. But if you're using your newfound veganism as a reason to explore cooking and eating to a new level, then you will probably want to expand your use of commonly cooked foods like rice. I could write a whole chapter on rice, the differences between them, and what they are best suited to, but I won't. What I will mention, however, is that while a good quality long-grain rice, like basmati, is a great all-rounder, make sure you try a great risotto, sushi or paella version for making these dishes, and for the most nutritional benefit consider trying out wholegrain rice.

Soya chunks and mince

If you quite like meat replacements, but you are trying to stick to a budget, bags of dried soya pieces are a gift from the universe. You can buy chunks, which are great for a curry, mince, which is just fabulous in a bolognese or chilli, and if you pop to an East Asian supermarket, you will find all kinds of 'ribs', 'chicken pieces' and other interesting versions, usually from Vietnam. They are really easy to use, you just soak them in boiling water or stock for a few minutes, then squeeze out the liquid and pop them into your dish. I find that these work best in saucy meals, like curries or stews, where they soak up whatever delicious liquid is in your pan. They don't fry so well, because they're wet.

Spices and seasonings

These are items that I think everybody should have a cupboard full of, vegan or not. For vegans in particular, spices are important for making simple foods like tofu, sweet potatoes, soya chunks, etc., all very tasty. But they are also full of their own health-promoting properties. If you aren't very confident with spices, perhaps start with a ready-mixed curry powder, then start experimenting. Here is a list of must-haves for a vegan-friendly cupboard:

- turmeric
- paprika (smoked and sweet are great, too)
- cumin (ground and seeds)
- ground coriander
- onion powder
- garlic powder
- kala namak (an eggy tasting black salt)

Stock cubes

To be honest, I think stock cubes are a must for any store cupboard, and vegetable stock is so readily available (just make sure it doesn't contain any lactose, because I have seen this, albeit rarely). The reason why stock cubes are mentioned here is because there are now some great vegan 'chicken' and 'beef' style stocks on the market, which can really enhance your dishes, and even make them taste more like old familiar meals that you might have enjoyed before transitioning. Be sure to check out the stock section at your local super-market.

Tofu

Tofu is often laughed at by vegan-sceptics, but every vegan will tell you, that if you don't like tofu, then you haven't had it cooked properly for you. It's not just for vegans, and has been used in many parts of Asia for a long, long time as part of an omnivorous diet, as well as for replacing meat. Tofu is made from soya beans, and as such is just full of fantastic nutritious benefits. It's also really tasty and so, so versatile. It comes in many different forms, so do some exploring and try them all. The staples in our house are silken tofu, which we use for scramble, chocolate pudding and creamy sauces, and we always have a pack of extra-firm tofu in the fridge for frying up nice and crispy with noodles and rice.

Vinegars

Good quality vinegar is a really important staple in your kitchen. I like a variety, including apple cider (with the mother, for the added probiotic benefits), and a sherry vinegar for making delicious salad dressing. Rice wine vinegar is also great for East Asian dishes.

What about Non-food Items?

When thinking about veganism, it's often easy to forget that it is more than just a diet, but veganism does apply to every-thing humans consume and use. When thinking about our patterns of buying and use of resources, we really do need to consider every-thing that's in our households, not just what we're eating.

Clothing

Leather

Even before I went vegan, I remember starting to feel very guilty about my leather shoes. It's another one of those products that we just don't think about a great deal. But when you consider what you are using, it really does feel barbaric. The skin of another, once liv-ing, breathing being, on your feet, in a day and age when there are plenty of alternatives. Then you become vegan and you stop wearing leather shoes, and soon realise that there are lots of other fabrics that also need to be avoided.

Silk

I know it's not used very commonly because of the cost, but silk is a rather cruel fabric. It's made from silk worms, the caterpillars of a type of moth. They use the protein fibre fibroin to weave their cocoons, but not only is silk exploitative because it utilises a substance that other creatures require for their own means, the process of obtaining this from the worms is rather brutal. The worms are bred in captivity, and once they begin making their cocoons, they are dissolved in boiling water so that their fibroin fibres can be extracted.

Wool

Wool is taken from the coats of sheep, often seemingly harmlessly, because they are not slaughtered for this purpose. However, the shearing process is often stressful and painful, with injuries occurring. It is also important to know, however, that around one third of wool comes from lambs that have been slaughtered for meat,[359] and that all sheep, whether they are bred for wool or not, will eventually be killed for their meat. 'Lambswool' comes from babies that are either being slaughtered at a very young age, or being sheared for the very first time, and is marketed as being more special because of its softness. But, with this comes the additional sadness of this product coming from mere babies.

As well as the considerations around the cruelty of wool, and how it's tied up with slaughter of sheep for meat, there are also implications for the environment and our health. Firstly, pesticides are used to remove bugs from the sheep, and these are harmful to human health and the environment.[360, 361] Then there are the additional environmental concerns about the effects of grazing sheep on ecosystems, and the subsequent reduction in biodiversity. These effects and the issue of carbon emissions are discussed in more detail in the 'Vegan for the Planet' chapter, but we need to understand how there isn't just one problem of farming sheep for meat or wool; it's all linked, and it's all problematic.

Cashmere, mohair and pashmina

These are other types of wool, but they come from goats. Again, some of this comes from slaughtered goats, and it can take 4–6 goats to make just one sweater. Because most of this type of wool comes from Asia, it is important to note the environmental effects of transporting the produce, as well as the local effects.[362]

Angora

Angora is the hair of Angora rabbits, who are bred in captivity and have their hair collected rather brutally. It is plucked whilst the rabbits are alert and awake, which, as you can probably imagine, is a painful experience. Angora rabbits are also bred very similarly to caged hens, living a miserable life in cramped quarters.

Other woolly fabrics

Many animals are used for their wool, and none of the practices for removing this hair is particularly humane or kind. Fabrics to watch out for include those made from alpaca, llama and camel, which all involve cruel ways of harvesting the hair, but some also have particularly high costs for the environment.

Felt can also catch you out. Although many felted fabrics are made from synthetic yarns, real wool is traditionally used for felts.

Fur

Fur describes the skin of an animal, and isn't just a vegan issue. I say this because while some fabrics we have discussed here could be argued to be 'by-products' (albeit questionably), fur most definitely isn't one of these. Fur requires the slaughter and skinning of animals such as mink, otters, beavers, coyote, and even bears. Thankfully, at least in the UK, fur is far less fashionable than it used to be, with many people decrying its use, even if they aren't vegan. However, tens of millions of animals around the world are still raised and killed for their skins. They are bred in miserable, cramped conditions, and sadly skinning animals alive isn't unheard of. Some wild animals are even trapped and killed for their skins.

Whilst real fur usually needs to be sought out and purchased from specialist sellers, it is easy to be duped into buying items which have small amounts of fur included in them, for example in the bobble of a woolly hat. It's important to check items that look like they contain fur to make sure it is just a synthetic 'faux' fur.

Feathers

Feathers aren't just used for flamboyant items like feather boas. They can be found in something as simple as the lining of your warm coat, which you hadn't really thought about, or the filling for your plump pillows. Once again, feathers are often seen as a by-product from the poultry industry, but apart from the fact that anybody avoiding animal exploitation probably wouldn't feel comfortable wrapping themselves in the plumage of an animal who has been slaughtered, feathers often come from animals who are kept alive longer than they usually would have been, just for the purpose of being plucked.

What are the alternatives?

There are lots of arguments from non-vegans that we might be responsible for more environmental damage because of the use of synthetic fabrics instead of more natural animal-derived fibres and fabrics. This could be true, but we don't need to rely on synthetics. We could use cottons, bamboo, hemp and linen, and there are also some really innovative materials around like lyocell made from wood pulp, and vegan leathers made from fruit skins. And whilst we know that synthetic fibres can be terrible for the environment, animal-derived fabrics aren't always better, because the farming of the animals that provide these have detrimental effects on local environments and the climate. Of course an option could be to use pre-loved items made from leather and wool, but many vegans don't feel comfortable wearing the skin of an animal once they have become conscious of how their clothing came to be, and the suffering that it was associated with. That choice would be yours, alone, to make. But there are more and more great, ethical choices coming onto the market.

Cleaning Products

The main issue that makes cleaning products non-vegan is the fact that they may be tested on animals. But not everything is, and you can often get 'leaping bunny' certified cruelty-free items in most supermarkets. Many of these are the supermarket's own brand, but others which are known to be cruelty-free include Ecover, Ecozone, Astonish and Method.

As far as I am aware, there aren't that many non-vegan ingredients in cleaning products, but the ones you want to consider are beeswax in items like furniture polish, and honey.

Beauty Products

Cruelty-free

As with household and cleaning items, one major problem with beauty items is that they are often tested on animals, making them cruel, and therefore non-vegan even when they are labelled as 'vegan friendly' just because they don't contain any animal-derived products. But you really shouldn't be able to call a product vegan when animals have been used and exploited in the production of that item. So make sure that any products are also labelled as cruelty-free, preferably with the 'leaping bunny' logo as well as being marked vegan. If something doesn't have leaping bunny certification, to make sure it really is cruelty-free, you need to make sure that the company doesn't sell their items in China, because their laws dictate that all beauty items have to be animal-tested before sale there. For this reason, a company that really cares about animal cruelty will not sell their items in China.

Beeswax and honey

As for non-vegan ingredients in beauty products, the culprits are similar to those in household items. Beeswax often makes an appearance, and before veganism became popular, I found it very difficult to find a decent mascara, because many of them rely on beeswax for the right texture. Again, honey might be found in creams and lotions.

Cochineal

You need to be careful of non-vegan colourings, like cochineal (E120, see the plant-based pitfalls chapter for more information) in items that are pigmented red.

Lanolin

Another animal-derived ingredient is lanolin, a fatty substance from sheep's wool, which is often found in moisturisers.

Shellac

Shellac, a glossy substance made from crushed beetles, is found in nail polish, hairspray, mascara and some moisturisers. Interestingly, the gel nail system named 'Shellac' doesn't actually contain the stuff from insects, but neither is it vegan because it's not cruelty-free.

Animal hair

Animal hairs can be found in false eyelashes and make up brushes, but many are also made from good quality synthetic substances.

Collagen

This is a substance made from the connective tissues of animals, and is often found in skin products.

Medication

As a vegan doctor, this is an area of veganism that has always in-terested me. Officially, medications are exempt from the philosophy, with The Vegan Society reminding us that 'the definition of veganism recognises that it is not always possible or practicable to avoid animal use in a non-vegan world. Sometimes, you may have no alternative to medication manufactured using animal products'. The animal products that they are eluding to are usually gelatine and lactose, which are used as fillers in medications. We also have to remember that even when medications don't contain these, they still can't be called vegan, because they all must be tested on animals, as per UK law.

There are sometimes safe ways around some of these issues, however. Remembering that they still will have been tested on animals, we can find versions of some medications that don't contain animals products. These are usually easier to access when they are items that can be bought over the counter, rather than prescribed medications, because you don't have gate-keeping doctors to get past. So let's take a look at some of the options.

Paracetamol

Paracetamol tablets usually contain lactose, the same as other white, powdery tablets. But there are a couple of brands which don't contain this, and they can be found at my website.[363] These are not always readily available, so you might want to consider a different way to take it, and one way of doing so is to buy soluble paracetamol, or even children's liquid paracetamol.

Ibuprofen

This is usually found in tablet or capsule form, with the former containing lactose, and the latter containing gelatine. Again, this can be bought as a children's formulation, which is a liquid, so free from both animal ingredients.

Antihistamines

Hay fever medications, whilst can also be purchased in a liquid form intended for children, can also be avoided by using other items that are great at targeting the individual symptoms of hay fever. For example, for itchy eyes there are some great eye drops and sprays on the market which target irritation and dryness. For nasal congestion and sneezing you can buy nasal sprays which contain steroids to combat the nasal symptoms of hay fever.

For prescribed medications, you won't really get a say in what your doctor prescribes for you, in terms of which brand or formulation of the medication you both agree on together. As we've already discussed, medication is exempt from the philosophy of veganism, and the NHS is in financial dire straits. So I never recommend demanding a liquid version of prescribed medication from your GP; as well as it being so expensive that if we all did it we would break the NHS, I also think it could risk damaging your relationship with your doctor, because they will find it difficult to manage your expectations and do the right thing. If you have a good rapport with your GP, I think it might be worth asking if there is a liquid version available to you, because sometimes there is one which isn't going to break the bank. So, it's worth asking the question, but you can't demand a 'vegan' version.

Entertainment

Zoos and circuses

Animals are used in lots of places where they are exploited for fun. The most obvious one in the UK is zoos. Whilst many people will argue that zoos do conservation work and offer education about wildlife, the counter-argument is that we do not need to keep these animals captive and away from their natural habitats in order to do either of these things. One of the principles which vegans live by, is that humans are not superior to any other animal, nor are our needs greater than those of other species. Most vegans will, therefore, believe that zoos are unethical places, holding animals captive against their will.

Circuses don't really have any feasible arguments to support their use of animals for entertainment. They have animals which have been trained to perform tricks, and the only way to train an animal is by force. They are usually beaten, so it's no surprise when these animals turn on their trainers and attack them. Where zoos do offer some benefits like conservation, circuses are purely for entertainment. However, many circuses are now animal-free, so you can still attend and enjoy the circus with your family, without paying for and partaking in animal cruelty.

Sport

Horses and greyhounds are forced to race, and apart from the painful injuries of the racing itself, we also need to consider the way in which these animals are bred and then slaughtered when they are no longer needed. And we're not just talking about shooting horses with awful racing injuries because it's the easiest and least expensive way to manage them, but many horses are sent to the abattoir to be killed for meat. In 2022, over 2000 racehorses in England and Ireland were killed for the meat industry.[364]

Holidays

Sometimes going on holiday can mean confronting situations that we're not faced with at home. Animal welfare laws vary around the world, and whilst most of the animal abuse in the UK is hidden behind walls, it's sometimes far more apparent when you are travelling overseas. This can mean seeing the mistreatment of animals for the entertainment of tourists. It can look like rides being offered to you on donkeys and horses, but let's not forget that this happens here in the UK, too. Further afield you might be offered a ride on an elephant or a camel, and it might seem rather exiting. But, please remember that these animals are often beaten during their training, treated dreadfully, and are not here for our entertainment. Sadly, it's also not unusual to see monkeys, snakes and other animals being used to make tourists laugh, and earn the locals a small income, but it's important to remember that they are wild animals, and are not here to serve us.

21

A Typical Day

I am going to give you an example of what a typical day looks like for me, in terms of eating and drinking, because I know that making changes that are so far from what you are currently doing can mean that visualising what life might look like is difficult. I've split my meals, snacks and drinks into 'ideal day' choices and 'busy day' choices. I don't like generalising too much with foods, but I know that, for me, there are less desirable choices, and more desirable choices, and that these won't be the same for everyone. An ideal choice for me is one that is closer to whole-food plant-based, but as long as everything that goes into my body is vegan, at the end of the day I'll feel happy. Please don't read my 'ideal' or 'busy' choices as any kind of judgement on the food, or on anybody else who makes different food choices from me. This is just how I like to eat.

Breakfast

Ideal day

When I've got plenty of time, I like to start with a cafetiere of fresh coffee. I often don't eat until later in the morning, but if I'm really hungry I will have a slice of wholemeal toast with peanut butter or maybe a bowl of muesli with soya milk. At the weekend, when we have time, we might make something like my Big Breakfast recipe, or at least just a tofu scramble on toast.

Busy day

On a busy day, my food situation is usually the same, but I'll be rushing and have an instant coffee instead of fresh. If it's the weekend and we're having a treat, we might have some vegan pastries, like perhaps some ready-to-bake pain au chocolat. Most ready-to-bake pastries that are readily found in many supermarkets are vegan, which is super convenient when you are short of time in the mornings.

Mid-morning Snack

Ideal day

When I'm working, I always take a small box of nuts and fruits with me. It will usually contain cashews, almonds, pecans, walnuts, peanuts and Brazil nuts, with dates or figs and dried apricots. Sometimes I'll sprinkle mixed seeds on there, too. I make sure I've got a good supply of fresh fruits, as well, with bananas, apples and oranges always in our fruit bowl.

Busy day

If I'm in a rush, I won't have had time to get my usual snack, so I might throw a raw fruit and nut bar (something like the Nakd brand) or an oat Graze bar into my bag, but I've usually got a piece of fresh fruit, too. I might have a rare treat of a biscuit with a cup of tea. The usual culprits, because they are vegan and readily available, are HobNobs, chocolate bourbons, or Biscoff. But as these don't offer too much in the way of nutritional value, I don't eat them very often.

Lunch

Ideal day

In the warmer weather I will try to make a big salad for my midday meal. I'll have the usual suspects of salad leaves, tomatoes, cucumber and tomatoes, but I'll often grate in some apple or carrot, and perhaps add a spoonful of capers, pickles or sauerkraut. I might throw in lentils, beans or tofu for some extra protein, and I'll make a nice dressing with herbs, oil and vinegar (see my recipes), or in a rush I'll just drizzle with extra virgin olive oil. I always try to top my salads with a good sprinkle of mixed seeds. In the cooler weather I'll make a soup with lots of vegetables and red lentils. Very often, I've got a portion of whatever was left over from last night's dinner.

Busy day

If I have forgotten to bring something from home, when I'm working I might get some bread and houmous from the supermarket, or maybe I'll buy some Quorn slices, vegan mayo if it's available, and salad, and make a quick sandwich. It's rare that I buy a take away these days, but if I do, it's usually sushi or a poke bowl. Occasionally if I'm in a huge rush, a Gregg's vegan sausage roll, or a supermarket sandwich will fill a gap until I can get something more nutritious into me.

Evening Meal

Ideal day

I usually batch cook and make enough for a few nights. This means that in a bind, I've usually got something good to eat in the fridge. My evening meal is usually something I've included in this book – either a curry, a lasagne, a rice dish or casserole. We have recently discovered a vegan company that makes meal kits, so we have a few of these delivered each week. They are whole-food, all entirely vegan, and very tasty. Perfect for a busy day! After dinner I do usually fancy something sweet, so I'll try to make it dried fruits, or a little bit of dark chocolate.When I've had the time and inclination, I sometimes have a tofu chocolate pudding in the fridge, which is a lovely hit of rich chocolate, with the added bonus of being nutritious and filling. Be sure to find the recipe for this one later in the book.

Busy day

So you might be thinking that my 'busy day' choices don't look too bad at all. But it's usually the evenings where I'll end up eating in a pattern that I feel isn't as healthy for me as I would like. If I haven't got any good batch-cooked food left in the fridge, then I might make some instant noodles with soya chicken pieces and a quick spicy sauce made with gochujang and soy sauce, or maybe I'll grab a take away. Sometimes this is delicious noodles or fried rice, or perhaps a curry from our favourite Sri Lankan place. Sometimes though, it is a burger and chips. Anywhere that serves Beyond Meat patties is a hit with us. I just try not to make it too often. If I'm craving a sugar hit in the evening, and my dried fruit or dark chocolate hasn't hit the spot, then I might have a cheeky Gü pot. They make delicious vegan cheesecakes, but they're definitely not for every day! Sometimes if I've got nothing in, I'll whip up a vegan mug cake using one of many online recipes.

Before Bed Drink

Ideal day

Once I'm able to wind down and do a bit of writing, I like to relax with a drink. I'll make some hot soya milk and have either cacao, carob or malt extract in it, or any combination of those, depending on what I'm in the mood for. If I don't have those things in, then I might have a decaf breakfast tea or a camomile tea.

Busy day

As you know, I don't drink alcohol any more, but sometimes, especially when the weather is nice, I still fancy a hit of something cold and sparking. So I'll have a chilled tonic water, or an alcohol-free lager when I'm unwinding and watching something on the TV.

22

Hints and Tips

Pack your nutrition in

I've mentioned that vegans often do much better than people who are omnivorous, just because we're thinking about our nutrition so much more. For me, this is because it's always on my mind since I started writing about nutrition and because I have children, but I'm often finding ways to pack as much nutrition into each meal as I can. This is what we should all be doing, really. Not only can you rest easy knowing that you're getting as much of the good stuff as possible, but you are also likely to feel fuller for longer when you pack high-protein, high-fibre foods into every dish.

One way I try to do this is to just empty a can of beans into a meal. For example, my Chick'n & Mushroom Pie in the recipes section once started off with vegan fake chicken pieces, but it now has tofu and a can of cannelini beans in. Because it's a creamy dish, you could pop a spoonful of nutritional yeast in, and some ground flaxseed. I also like sprinkling seeds on everything, from soups and salads, to my fried rice and even fruit and yoghurt.

Pack something to eat

Most places have something for vegans to eat. Even if that is just a plate of chips or a bag of salted crisps and a banana. But I got really fed up of living like this, especially when I also had disappointed kids to think about. So I usually take a delicious sandwich on a long trip, or a box of nuts and dried fruit to a meeting. If we're going somewhere the kids are likely to be getting a treat that they won't be able to eat, then I pack a vegan cake or biscuit, or even a bag of sweets if it's appropriate for where we're going. It saves a lot of grumbling bellies and disappointed little ones.

Get online

I mentioned finding your tribe in the 'What Should I Do First?' section, so I won't repeat myself too much here. What I will say though, is join as many vegan groups and follow as many vegan pages as you can. You can always leave if any of them aren't your vibe, but the more you're exposed to veganism, the more normal it will feel. There are also some brilliant recipe creators on TikTok and Instagram, so just save everything you see on there and give some of them a try.

Explore

When I became vegan in 2017, I felt a little bit sorry for myself. Whilst I was making a change that I knew I had to, I wasn't excited at first. I was worried about failure, and mostly about missing the foods that I knew. But what I soon found out was that I wasn't missing out on anything at all. In fact, I was opening up my culinary world to a whole host of foods and ingredients that I'd never tasted or cooked with before. Obviously, any omnivore could also explore these ingredients, but it's not until we're forced to become a bit imaginative about our cooking that we go looking for these things. Make sure you get brave and try lots of different things that you wouldn't have done before.

Forgive yourself

You're going to make mistakes and slip up. It might even take a few resets to get veganism to really stick for you. But that's OK. You're headed in the right direction. Society is set up for omnivores, so starting a new lifestyle which might seem to go against everything that we're taught, shown and sold isn't going to be easy. But it's very doable and you absolutely can do this.

Meet everyone with compassion

We have discussed how veganism is about compassion at its core, whether it is compassion for the animals, for the planet, or our own body and health, but we often forget about how we treat other human beings. I did discuss this a little in the 'Vegan for Social Justice' chapter, but I would suggest that we consider even those who don't appear to be affected by our food choices or lifestyles. What I mean is thinking about our response to those who don't understand or accept our choice to be vegan. Not everybody will understand, and some people may even treat you with aggression about your decision to follow a vegan lifestyle. But I honestly believe that even those people should be treated kindly. People don't know what they don't know, so while you have opened your eyes and your mind, most other people will still be living under the illusion that animals are here for us to use and consume, that they are not harmed or hurt by the animal agriculture industry, or at worst that it doesn't matter how we treat animals.

We've all been programmed to believe that we are superior to other animals, and as such we can do as we wish with them. It takes big change in your thinking and in your actions to get to the point where you can begin living a kinder life, and most people haven't made those connections yet. So I believe that, until they do, we should be kind to them. Your compassion and love for those people who judge your choices badly, or laugh at you for being vegan, is only going to have beneficial effects. Positivity is infectious. Even the most anti-vegan person might find themselves questioning whether veganism is worth a try when they see the goodness oozing out of vegans, rather than being confronted with aggression. We also have to bear in mind that once we have declared that veganism is right and true, you are admitting that everything that has gone before in your life was wrong, and as such, your lifestyle implies that everybody else is partaking in unethical practices – and no one enjoys being criticised.

Read

There are lots of great books and blogs on veganism. When I have made any big change in my life, whether it was having children, stopping drinking alcohol, or going vegan, I gathered as much information about it as I could, and consumed it all until I understood everything about it and my thinking switched. Yes, I am autistic, so these things becoming my special interest might have something to do with it. But, honestly, immersing myself in ideas that were aligned with where I wanted to be, made it all just feel so much more 'normal'.

RECIPES

Introduction

Now you've read about all the reasons why we should be aiming to live a plant-rich life, and I've reassured you that maintaining healthy nutrition is simple on a vegan diet once you understand what you need. I've given you tips on how to get started, and helped you with your shopping list. So the only thing left for me to do is to share some delicious recipes to set you on your way.

This is a collection of recipes which have come from my own kitchen. Some have been handed down, either fully or in part, from my mum and my nanna, who both cooked delicious meals for me when I was growing up. My mum still does! Others I have developed in a bid to have a veganised version of something I loved before.

I've split them into Breakfast and Snacks, Soups and Starters, Main Courses, and Sides and Salads. Of course you can eat any of them any which way you like, but some of them go particularly well together. There's just one pudding, but it's a good one.

I'm pretty relaxed when I am cooking, and it took quite a lot of discipline to write down proper measurements. As such, when you're cooking my recipes, you should feel free to be as relaxed as I am, and change around ingredients as you wish. If you want a different bean in your casserole, or a different bunch of veggies in your fried rice, then go ahead. You could sub vegan chick'n pieces for mushrooms in the stroganoff, or put rice noodles in the curried broth to keep it gluten free. I'll try to let you know if a dish is gluten free, or how to adapt it to make it so.

The main thing is to have fun, enjoy cooking, and more importantly, enjoy eating!

Notes

Oil: Where I've just written oil, that's usually because it's to be used for frying, so use your preferred cooking oil. I know it's a contentious topic these days! I still use rapeseed oil for cooking, as it's only in small quantities, and the omega-3 we're gaining from it is beneficial for us as a family. If I specify another oil, that's because it's important in the recipe for a particular flavour or nutrient profile.

Stock: Where I have recommended a particular style of stock (e.g. vegan chicken or beef), this is because that flavour suits that recipe. I tend to use Oxo 'meat-free' (in the yellow box for chicken style and the red box for beef style), but you can sub any vegan stock you prefer.

Plant milks: We use barista oat milk in our house, particularly on the kids' cereal, or for their drinks. We chose this to use for our family because of the slightly higher fat content which made it suitable for a toddler who wasn't having breast milk any more. I am finding myself moving towards soya milk at the moment, for reasons I've discussed in the 'Vegan for Health' section, so this usually gets used in my cooking. Most plant milks, unless they have a strong flavour, will work well in the majority of the recipes that call for milk. But bear in mind that if it isn't fortified with calcium, vitamin D, iodine and B12, then you won't have the same nutrient profile that I may have mentioned at the beginning of the recipe.

Breakfast and Snacks

The Big Breakfast

(Tofu scramble and avocado mash on toast with Mediterranean tomatoes and black pepper mushrooms)

This isn't called 'Big Breakfast' for nothing! It's a big, nutritious breakfast or brunch that will set you up for the day. You might want to cook this on a weekend though, as all the different components do take a little time to prepare. This recipe serves 2 people, and is scrumptious and full of goodness. It can be made gluten free with the right toast.

Tofu scramble

Ingredients:

- 1 pack of silken tofu
- 1 small red onion, finely chopped

- 1 small green chilli, chopped (use half if you don't want this to be spicy)
- ½ tsp of turmeric
- ½ tsp of kala namak (black salt) – if you can't find this, leave it out and just season with regular table salt, but you will be missing that eggy flavour
- 1–2 tsp of nutritional yeast flakes
- A pinch of coarsely ground black pepper
- Oil for cooking

Method:

1. Heat the oil in a frying pan, and sauté the onion and chilli until softened. Don't let the onion brown.
2. Add the turmeric and kala namak and stir it through before adding in the tofu. Break it up with your spoon into small pieces whilst stirring so it gets covered in the turmeric and kala namak. Don't worry if it continues breaking up, this makes it more like the texture of scrambled egg.
3. Stir the nutritional yeast through the mixture and finish with a sprinkling of black pepper. Leave it to one side whilst you get on with the rest of the dish.

Avocado mash

Ingredients:

- 1 large ripe avocado
- A splash of extra virgin olive oil or cold-pressed rapeseed oil
- A pinch of freshly crushed black pepper
- A pinch of sea salt

Method:

1. Scoop the avocado from its skin, roughly chop and place it into a wide, shallow bowl.
2. Mash with the back of a fork until soft, then add the oil, salt and pepper, and continue mashing until it's smooth.
3. If you have other parts of the recipe to prepare, put the avocado stone into the bowl with the mash, and cover to prevent it from going brown.

Black pepper mushrooms

Ingredients:

- 250g carton of baby chestnut mushrooms, halved
- ¼ tsp ground black pepper
- Oil for cooking

Method:

1. Heat the oil in a frying pan over a medium heat
2. Add the mushrooms and sauté until softened, stirring so they don't brown too much. You can add more oil if the mushrooms are sticking to the pan, but be careful not to add too much, as mushrooms can act like little sponges.
3. Just before finishing, add the black pepper and stir through.

Mediterranean tomatoes

Ingredients:

- 1 carton of baby plum tomatoes
- A splash of extra virgin olive oil
- 1 sprig of fresh basil, roughly torn
- 1 clove garlic, roughly chopped
- A sprinkle of sea salt

Method:

1. Heat the olive oil over low-medium heat.
2. Add the whole tomatoes, chopped garlic and roughly torn basil leaves.
3. Gently sauté for 10 minutes or until the tomatoes have softened but are still whole.
4. Season to taste with salt.

Putting it all together

Other ingredients:

- 2 slices of toasted sourdough bread, or other vegan bread of your choice (gluten free if preferred or required)
- A pinch of paprika

Method:

1. Spread the avocado mash over the toast, sprinkle with a little paprika and slice them in half.
2. Place the pieces of avocado toast on 2 large plates, with a small gap between the two halves.
3. Put a mound of the tofu scramble in the middle of the plates between the toast halves.
4. Scatter the mushrooms and tomatoes around the plates, allowing some to fall onto the avocado toast and tofu scramble.

Banana and Chia Pancakes

This recipe makes around 10–12 small pancakes, perfect for little hands if you have any kids to feed. Do feel free to make fewer, large pancakes for the grown-ups, though. I find that these are a good way to use up very ripe bananas, and also to get some hidden fruit and seeds into my little ones.

Adding chia seeds provides a great dose of omega-3, as well as magnesium, iron and calcium. Add that to the calcium, B12 and vitamin D content of your fortified milk, and you've got one nutritious pancake on your hands!

Ingredients:

- 1 cup of plain flour
- 1 tsp of bicarbonate of soda
- 2 tbsp chia seeds
- 1 large ripe banana mashed
- 1 cup any plant milk
- ½ tsp vanilla extract
- 1 tsp apple cider vinegar
- Oil for cooking

Method:

1. In a batter jug or large mixing bowl, combine the flour, bicarb and chia seeds.

2. In another bowl, thoroughly mash the banana, then combine well with the milk, apple cider vinegar, and vanilla extract.
3. Transfer the banana mixture to the batter jug, and mix the dry and wet ingredients together thoroughly.
4. Pop a splash of oil in a large frying pan and put it over a medium heat. Once the oil is hot enough, pour small batches of the mixture into the hot oil. Allow them to cook for 1–2 minutes until lightly browned and crisp, then flip with a slotted spatula.
5. Cook for the same amount of time on the other side until they are also brown and crispy.
6. Remove from the pan and place on a clean absorbent towel to remove excess oil, then serve as they are or with berries and a dollop of thick soya yoghurt.

Alternative Flavours

Add a handful of blueberries instead of (or as well as) banana and chia seeds for an antioxidant boost.

Add a heaped tablespoon of peanut butter to your wet mixture – it goes well with banana, and adds a dose of healthy fat and extra vitamins.

Good quality dark cholocate chips make a nice addition for a treat. (Be sure to sprinkle these on after you've transferred the batter to the frying pan and the pancake has started cooking, otherwise they can sink through to the pan and burn on contact.)

Avocado and Smoky Mushrooms on Toast

So if you haven't got time (or the stomach space) for the Big Breakfast, this lighter option serves two as a great brunch or breakfast. It contains good fats in the avocado and cold-pressed rapeseed oil, and can be whipped up in less than half an hour.

Keep this gluten free with tamari instead of soy sauce, and serve it on gluten-free toast.

Ingredients:

- 500g chestnut mushrooms, thickly sliced
- 2 tbsp of soy sauce
- 2 tbsp of maple syrup
- 2 tsp of smoked paprika
- 2 large, ripe avocado, skin and stone removed, and cut into large pieces
- 2 tsp of cold-pressed rapeseed oil
- Cracked black pepper for seasoning
- Oil for cooking
- 4 slices of sourdough

Method:

1. Heat a splash of oil in a frying pan, then throw in the sliced mushrooms. Keep stirring to make sure they cook evenly. Fry for around 5–10 minutes.

2. While the mushrooms are cooking mix the soy sauce, maple syrup and smoked paprika in a small bowl.

3. In another bowl, mash the avocado with a fork, then add the rapeseed oil and continue mashing and mixing until the avocado is nice and smooth, whilst toasting your bread.

4. Pour the soy, maple and paprika mix into the pan, stir well and simmer for a few minutes until the sauce has all been absorbed.

5. Take the mushrooms off the heat and start building your dish. Spread the avocado thickly onto each slice of toast, then place onto two plates. Put a mound of mushrooms on top of each slice of bread, and finish with a twist of fresh black pepper.

I sometimes like to top this dish with a sprinkle of mixed seeds for extra crunch and nutrition.

C ourgette Fritters

I've had a few great versions of courgette fritters, but I came up with this recipe after a visit back to my folks' house, where I was happily greeted with a lovely soup accompanied by some fantastic fritters made with courgettes from their garden.

This recipe makes around 10 fritters depending on how much batter you heap into the pan each time, but it easily serves 4 as a starter or light lunch, more for a snack.

Ingredients:

(For the fritters)

- 2 large courgettes, grated
- 2 spring onions, finely sliced
- 1 heaped tbsp of fresh mint, chopped
- 1 heaped tbsp of fresh dill, chopped
- 1 cup of plain flour
- 2 tsp of baking powder
- Oil for cooking
- Pinch of salt

(For the tzatziki dip)

- 1 cup of plain soya yoghurt
- 1 tbsp of fresh mint, chopped
- ½ large cucumber
- 1 tbsp of extra virgin olive oil
- Juice of half a lemon

Method:

1. Place the grated courgette into a colander lined with a clean tea towel. Sprinkle them with a little salt, rub the courgettes all over to coat them in the salt, and leave them for a few minutes.
2. Place the chopped herbs, spring onions, flour and baking powder in a large bowl and combine.
3. Squeeze the liquid out of the courgettes, twisting the towel around them to get every drop out, then put them in the bowl with the other ingredients.
4. Mix everything, making sure the courgettes are covered in the flour mixture and leave it to stand for 10 minutes.
5. Meanwhile, make your tzatziki. In a small bowl, mix together the yoghurt, mint, cucumber, lemon juice and olive oil. Leave it to one side while you get back to the fritters.
6. Heat a splash of oil in a shallow frying pan. When you come back to the courgette mixture, it should be sticky from the flour absorbing the liquid in the courgettes. Scoop a small amount of the batter, maybe a heaped tablespoon or so, roll it into a ball in your hands, and carefully place into the hot oil. Repeat three more times, then flatten each of the balls with the back of a spatula
7. Once the fritters have browned, flip them to cook the other side. Once they have turned brown and crispy, transfer them

to a plate topped with a clean absorbent towel to remove excess oil. Repeat the process until you've used all of your courgette mixture up.

8. Serve the fritters warm with a side of creamy tzatziki.

Houmous

I know that houmous is so easy to buy, but there's something special about making it just to your own taste. It's also a great back up dish when you need a quick lunch or starter, especially when there are little people in the house. I've never known a vegan kiddo who doesn't like houmous!

As always, this houmous is gluten-free.

Ingredients:

- 1 tin of chickpeas in water – drained, but keep the aquafaba
- Juice of 1 lemon
- ½ cup of tahini
- ½ cup of extra virgin olive oil
- 2 garlic cloves roughly chopped
- Salt to taste

Method:

1. Drain the chickpeas, but keep the aquafaba.
2. Add the chickpeas, half of the lemon juice, tahini, oil, garlic and half a cup of the aquafaba to a high speed blender. Don't worry too much if your blender isn't super fast, but bear in mind that the faster it is, the smoother your houmous will be. Blend it for a minute, stopping and scraping the sides down

if necessary. If it's too stiff to continue blending, add another tablespoon of aquafaba and try again.

3. Once you've got a smooth houmous, stop blending and, using a clean spoon, have a taste. If it's not tangy enough, add another tablespoon of lemon juice, or more if you wish. Add salt to taste. If you would like it a little looser and smoother, add another tablespoon of aquafaba.

4. Blend again, taste again, and repeat as above until you've got the taste and consistency right for you.

Alternative Flavours

Roasted red pepper: When you're blending for the first time, add 1 or 2 roasted red peppers from a jar for a red pepper houmous.

Lemon and coriander: Add the juice of the whole lemon juice and a tablespoon or two of chopped, fresh coriander.

Sweet potato: Blend in a few pieces of roasted sweet potato, leaving out the lemon juice.

Mediterranean Meatloaf

I had my toddler in mind when I first made this recipe. He was going through a phase of fussy eating, but I knew that vegan sausages always went down well. To provide him with a bit of variety, but keeping 'safe foods' in mind, I decided to make his beloved sausages into something a little more interesting, with a change in flavour and texture for variety. But it turned out that the whole family enjoyed this 'meatloaf'!

This is usually one of my batch-cooked mega dishes! It serves 8–10, or will keep in the fridge for a few days, so you can go back to it. It's really tasty when slices are pan-fried in a little oil to crisp up the outside.

Ingredients:

- 2 packs of vegan sausages – I use Richmond's for this recipe. You can use others, but you need something like a traditional sausage with a skin and sausage 'meat' on the inside
- 3 tbsp of sundried tomato paste
- 1 cup of white breadcrumbs
- 1 flax egg (see below)
- 1 tbsp of dried oregano or mixed Italian herbs
- 1 cup of vegan stock – I like beef-style cubes for this recipe

Method:

1. Heat the oven to 180C and line a loaf tin with baking paper.
2. Prepare your flax egg as per the instructions below.
3. Remove the skin from the sausages, and discard them. Place the contents into a large mixing bowl and break them up with the back of a fork or a wooden spoon.
4. Pour the stock, tomato paste and herbs into the bowl with the sausage 'meat' and use a potato masher to break the 'meat' up further and combine it with the other ingredients.
5. Add the breadcrumbs and flax egg to the bowl, and mix well.
6. Transfer the mixture into the paper-lined loaf tin and press it down well into all of the corners, and smooth the top down.
7. Place the loaf tin onto a baking tray, and put it in the middle of the oven for 30 minutes.
8. Remove the loaf from the oven, and once this has cooled enough to handle, pull at the edges of the paper to lift the loaf out of the tin. Tip it upside down on a chopping board, and once it has cooled a bit more slice it thickly.
9. Serve with mash, veg and gravy for a main meal, or salad for a light lunch. This also works really well sliced up and fried as a brunch or snack the following day, and a friend pointed out that it's far more sophisticated when served sliced and smothered in a delicious tomato sauce.

How to make a flax egg:

Mix 1 tablespoon of ground flaxseed with 3 tablespoons of water, and allow it to sit for 5–10 minutes until it turns into a gel.

Butter Bean Pate

This recipe came from my mum, and was another treat with which I was greeted at the door when I arrived on one of my visits. My parents live very far from where I am, in fact they live very far from many people! So to visit them, I have to take a trip of around 6 hours and I usually arrive tired and hungry. I think one of my enduring memories of my mum will be her in the kitchen preparing either the perfect vegan salad sandwich so it's fresh and ready just as we arrive, or serving something like this tasty dip, a warming soup, or nourishing courgette fritters.

This pate is naturally gluten-free.

Ingredients:

- 1 tin of butter beans, drained
- 1-inch piece of lemon rind, peeled with a potato peeler
- 1 clove of garlic, sliced
- 1 small sprig of fresh thyme
- ¼ cup of extra virgin olive oil
- Salt and black pepper to season

Method:

1. In a small pan, warm the olive oil, and place the garlic, thyme and lemon rind into it. Let it gently simmer for 10 minutes, but make sure not to let the garlic brown.
2. Tip the butter beans into a good, fast blender, and add the oil and garlic, but remove the lemon and thyme. Blend well until it is all smooth.
3. Serve with crusty bread, toast or crudités.

Japanese-Style Vegetable Pancakes

This is a quick, easy way to get a couple of portions of veg into your little ones, but it's also really delicious as a side dish to either a fried rice, or perhaps bibimbap. You can mix the selection of veggies up, but cabbage, carrot and spring onion work really well. Much like my banana and chia pancakes, this can also be made as small pancakes which are suitable for little hands, but I really like this as a large pancake which can be cut into individual portions and shared.

Ingredients:

- ½ medium savoy cabbage
- 2 large carrots
- 5 spring onions
- 1 cup of plain flour
- 1 cup of plant milk
- 1 tsp of kala namak
- Oil for frying

Method:

1. Shred the cabbage by removing the thick stalk and cutting into fine slices. Grate the carrots, and finely slice the spring onions into long, thin pieces.

2. In a large mixing bowl combine the flour and kala namak, then pour in the milk, whisking as you go to avoid lumps.

3. Add the vegetables to the batter and mix well to make sure that all the pieces of vegetable are coated in batter.

4. Put a splash of oil into a small, shallow frying pan and place it over a medium heat. Once hot, spoon around half of the pancake mixture to cover the bottom of the pan to around a 1cm thickness. Fry until the bottom is crispy and browned.

5. Take a slice/turner and run it around the edges of the pancake to make sure it's not stuck down, then gently run it under the bottom of the pancake. Take a heat resistant chopping board, or a flat oven tray and place it over the pan, holding it down with an oven-gloved hand, and flip the pan upside down, tipping the pancake onto the board. Pop the pan back onto the heat, and use the slice to slide the pancake back in to the pan, uncooked side down.

6. Fry for a further few minutes until the bottom is crisped and brown again.

7. Remove the pancake from the pan onto a clean absorbent towel to remove excess oil, then repeat the process until you have used up all the mix.

8. Cut each pancake into 6 slices and stack them all onto a serving plate. Serve with any main course of your choice, or drizzle in Sriracha mayo and enjoy as a delicious lunch.

Mango and Mint Summer Rolls

I love summer rolls. So much so that I'm often pushing the definition of a summer roll by stuffing whatever sandwich filling I fancy into a rice paper wrapper. But I'm pretty sure I'm allowed to call this version a summer roll!

These light, fresh rolls serve 4 as a starter, or two as a light lunch or snack. Although there isn't really any cooking for this recipe, it is a labour of love, as you need to soak each wrapper individually, then fill and assemble each roll one-by-one. Keep it gluten free with tamari instead of soy sauce, and you can make this a bit more filling by adding slices of fried tofu, or even a couple of slices of vegan deli 'chicken.'

Ingredients:

- 8 rice paper spring roll wrappers
- 2 cakes of rice vermicelli noodles, soaked or cooked as per the instructions on the packet
- 1 large mango, thinly sliced
- ½ large cucumber, seeds removed and julienned
- 4 spring onions, julienned
- 1 large carrot, peeled, then ribboned with a peeler
- 2 tbsp roughly chopped coriander
- 1 sprig of mint, leaves removed from the stalk and finely sliced
- 2 tbsp soy sauce

- 1 tbsp lime juice
- Sweet chilli sauce for dipping

Method:

1. Put all of the vegetables, mango, prepared noodles, herbs, soy sauce and lime juice into a large bowl. Toss well, covering everything in the sauce and juice.
2. Fill a large, shallow dish with hot water. I boil a kettle, then wait for it to cool a little. Make sure your chopping board is wiped clean, but damp.
3. Put a rice paper wrapper into the hot water for around 10–20 seconds until it is soft and pliable, then place it on the wet chopping board.
4. Put ⅛ of the noodle and veg mix into the centre of the wrap, making sure there is a little bit of everything in there.
5. This is how I fold them: bring the bottom of the wrapper up over the noodle mixture, quite tightly, but not pulling hard enough to rip it. Then bring in each side, overlapping it onto the bottom part so it sticks a little. I put my thumbs under the roll, and my fingers on top, and roll upwards, keeping some tension on and tucking in the contents with my fingers as I go.
6. Once the roll is finished, transfer it to a large plate, folded side down so that it stays stuck down, then start on the next one. Make sure to keep a bit of space between folded rolls, as they sometimes rip when they get stuck together. Repeat 7 more times, and enjoy dipped into sweet chilli sauce.

Sweetcorn and Coconut Soup

This creamy, warming soup serves 4 people. It is gently spiced with ginger and chilli, and just so comforting on an autumn day. Taking just 25–30 minutes to cook, this is a wonderfully quick and easy lunch. Depending on how you prefer your soup, you can blend it as much or as little as you like; when I'm feeling fancy, I pass a well-blended soup through a sieve to create a really silky finished product. But it's equally tasty with a bit of texture. This recipe is gluten free.

Ingredients:

- 4 cups of frozen or tinned sweetcorn
- 2 medium onions, thinly sliced
- 1 tin of coconut milk
- 1 litre of vegetable or chicken-style stock
- 2 green chillies, finely chopped
- 4 tbsp of garlic ginger paste
- Oil for cooking
- Salt and pepper to season

Method:

1. Heat a splash of oil in a large pan and add the sliced onion. Cook it for 5 minutes until softened and lightly browned.
2. Add the garlic-ginger paste and chilli, and cook for another 2 minutes.
3. Add the sweetcorn to the pan and stir well before pouring in the stock and coconut milk, and simmer for 10 minutes.
4. Allow the soup to cool, then transfer it to a food processor. Blend until the soup is smooth, and any visible pieces have gone. Add any seasoning to taste, and give it another whizz.
5. Pour into 4 bowls and enjoy.

Naked Dumplings

I have always been a fan of various forms of dumplings, both of eating them, and making them. Whilst some dumpling or wonton wrappers are suitable for vegans, others contain egg. You can make your own wrappers, but this can be very fiddly and time consuming. So for a quick, easy lunch, I just wrap my dumpling filling in a crisp lettuce leaf, which also adds a lovely crunch. If you're cooking gluten free, sub the soy sauce for tamari, and make sure to use a gluten-free version of hoisin sauce, which is readily available

This will serve 2 people as a snack or light lunch, or more if you are serving other small dishes alongside it.

Ingredients:

- 1 cup or around 75g of dried soya mince
- 1 medium onion or two shallots, finely chopped
- 2 cloves of garlic, finely chopped or crushed
- 1 inch piece of ginger, peeled and grated
- ½ tsp of dried chilli flakes
- ½ tsp of Chinese five spice
- 3 spring onions, finely sliced
- 3 tbsp of light soy sauce
- Oil for cooking
- 1 tbsp of toasted sesame oil
- 1 baby gem lettuce

- Hoisin sauce to serve

Method:

1. Rehydrate the soya mince by covering it in boiling water in a bowl, and leave it for 15 minutes. Then drain the water off in a sieve, and leave the soya mince in the sieve to cool down and dry out a bit.
2. Heat a splash of oil in a frying pan over a medium heat. Add the onion, and fry or 1–2 minutes until it starts to brown.
3. Add garlic, ginger, spices and chilli flakes, and turn the heat down a little. Stir it well so the garlic and spices don't burn. Fry for 1 minute until you can smell the garlic and five spice.
4. Add the rehydrated soya mince to the pan and stir fry for 3–4 minutes before adding the soy sauce and sesame oil and continuing to stir. Take the pan off the heat.
5. Cut the root off the lettuce and carefully separate the leaves so they retain their 'cup' shape. Try not to tear them. Discard the leaves that will be too small to fill (save them for a salad), and rinse and dry the leaves that you are going to use.
6. Spoon the mince mixture into lettuce leaves, top them with the sliced spring onions, and serve drizzled with a dash of hoisin sauce.

Sweet Potato and Sage Soup

Is there a better food combination than sweet potato and sage? I don't think so! And this delicious pairing is just perfect in a smooth, creamy soup on a cold day. This is a super easy lunch dish, taking no more than an hour, with very little prep to do. And it will feed a hungry family of four, with bread to dunk in, of course. As long as the stock you are using is gluten-free, so is the entire recipe.

Ingredients:

- 3 large sweet potatoes, peeled and cut into 1 inch pieces
- 2 sticks of celery, sliced
- 1 onion, chopped
- 2 large carrots, sliced
- 1 litre of vegetable stock
- 1 tbsp of dried sage
- Oil for cooking

Method:

1. Heat the oven to 180C and allow it to warm up whilst preparing your vegetables.

2. Place the chopped sweet potatoes into a large oven dish, toss in a tablespoon of oil, then cook in the middle of the oven for 45 minutes. Turn once during cooking.

3. While the potatoes are roasting, heat a tablespoon of oil in a large pan. Add the onion, celery and carrots, and fry over a medium heat for around 10 minutes until soft. Don't allow them to brown. Add the sage, then cook for a further five minutes, stirring occasionally.

4. Pour the stock into the pan, bring to the boil, then simmer for half an hour.

5. Once the sweet potatoes are cooked, add them to the pan, and allow it all to cool. Use a stick blender to blend into a smooth soup. You can also use a food processor for this.

6. Ladle into 4 bowls and serve with crusty bread for a warming meal.

Onion Bhaji

Sometimes the stars align, and you find something that's vegan, comforting, AND gluten free. That means that everybody can enjoy it. I've got gluten-free members of the family, so I just love being able to share recipes and product suggestions that fill the vegan and gluten-free criteria. Really, traditionally made onion bhaji should be gluten free, as they are made with gram flour – also known as chickpea flour. Unfortunately, this isn't always the case with supermarket bhaji. But who needs to buy them from the supermarket when this recipe is so easy to make, and even more delicious?

This makes 8–10 large bhaji. Enough for all the family to have at least 2 each!

Ingredients:

- ½ cup of gram flour
- 1 tsp of baking powder
- 1 tsp of fennel seeds
- 1 tsp of cumin seeds
- ½ tsp ground cumin
- ½ tsp of ground coriander
- 1 tsp of turmeric
- A generous pinch of salt
- ½ cup of water
- 1 large red onion, thinly sliced

- Oil for cooking (see details below)

Method:

1. Put the gram flour, spices, seeds, salt and baking powder into a large bowl and combine well.
2. Add the water and mix into a thick batter. Add the onions to the bowl, and mix everything together so that all the onions are covered.
3. In a deep frying pan or a saucepan, pour oil to a depth of around 3 cm. It needs to be enough to submerge the bottom half of a bhaji. Heat the oil over a high flame, and when you think it's hot enough, test it with a spot of batter. It should sizzle when you put it in.
4. Using a dessert spoon, put a few dollops of the onion batter mix into the oil. Leave enough space between the bhaji to turn them. The number you can cook in one go will depend on the size of your pan. Cook it for 4 or 5 minutes, until it starts to look brown and crispy. Then flip them over and cook them all for a further 2–3 minutes.
5. Use a slotted spoon to remove the bhaji from the pan, and place them on a plate covered with a clean absorbent towel to remove excess oil. Serve either with your favourite curry, or just as a delicious snack.

Simple Lentil Soup

I just threw this soup together, one day, when I was pregnant and suffering from morning sickness. Its simplicity turned out to be absolutely perfect for what I needed, so I immediately wrote it down, and it's been my go-to soup when I'm under the weather ever since. Despite being a very simple dish, it's rich in fibre, protein and iron, and it's an easy dish to prepare that suits all the family, even the gluten-free members.

Ingredients:

- 1 brown onion, finely chopped
- 2 garlic cloves, finely chopped
- 2 carrots sliced
- 1 cup of red lentils
- 1 litre of stock – I use vegan chicken-style, but vegetable will also do
- ½ tsp of dried sage
- ½ tsp of dried thyme
- Oil for cooking
- Pinch of white pepper for seasoning

Method:

1. Heat a splash of oil in a large pan over a medium heat. Add the onion and carrot and sauté them until they have softened.

Add the garlic, sage and thyme, and cook for a few more minutes.

2. Add the lentils and stock, and bring it to a boil before turning down the heat. Cover and simmer for 30 minutes.

3. Check the lentils are soft and can be broken up with a spoon. If so, they are cooked, if not give them another 5 minutes.

4. Add white pepper to taste, plus salt to taste. I often find that the stock cubes are plenty salty enough.

5. Once cooled, use a stick blender to blend to your desired consistency. I like this one quite smooth, and blending makes it lovely and creamy.

6. Serve with crusty buttered bread.

Scotch Broth

My mum used to make this for me when I was very little, and I especially loved it when I felt unwell. It's a really simple dish, but it's comforting and nutritious. It's a proper generational, hand-me down type dish; my mum had it made for her by her mother, she made it for me, and now I make it for my little ones when they're under the weather.

This will serve around 4 people. Feel free to play around with the combination of vegetables and grains. This version is just the way I prefer it. If you would like to keep it gluten-free, replace the barley with another suitable grain.

Ingredients:

- 1 large onion, thinly sliced
- 2 large carrots, thickly sliced – I leave the skin on for this recipe but feel free to peel them if you prefer
- 2 sticks of celery, thickly sliced
- 1 large potato, diced into large pieces – again, I leave the skin on, but feel free to peel them, if you prefer
- ½ cup of pearl barley
- 1 litre of vegan chicken-style stock
- 1 tsp of dried sage
- 1 tsp of dried thyme, or a sprig of fresh thyme if you have it

- 250g of soya mince – this is optional. You can leave out the meat replacement, if you prefer, and it still tastes great
- Oil for frying
- Salt and pepper to taste

Method:

1. Heat a splash of oil in a large, heavy pan over a medium heat. Add the soya mince and fry until crispy, then remove from the pan to a plate lined with a clean, absorbant towel to remove excess oil.
2. Add the onion, carrot and celery to the hot pan and fry gently for 5–7 minutes until the veggies are soft, but not brown.
3. Add the herbs, and cook for a further 2 minutes.
4. Pour in the pearl barley and stock, make sure everything is combined, and turn up the heat. Bring to a boil before reducing it back down to a simmer and leave it covered for half an hour.
5. Add the potatoes and mince and replace the lid. Cook for 20 minutes until the potatoes are soft enough to break with a fork.
6. Season and serve with crusty bread, or just as it is.

Vegetable Fried Rice

We have a fried rice most weeks. It's one of those dishes that can be thrown together quickly in between work, nursery and school runs, and chores. I prepare it in stages, boiling my rice in the morning before baby's lunchtime nap, then slice my veggies while she's having a snack, and do my final bit of cooking after the school run, just in time for dinner.

This serves 4, and is pretty versatile; you can switch the vegetables for whatever you've got in the fridge, or just to what you want to eat that evening. I tend to use basmati rice, as I find that the long grains suit being coated in the sauce, but other rices work well, and you can use different grains for various flavours of sauce. I sometimes like to add some vegan chicken-style pieces to my fried rice, but cubed tofu, tossed in seasoned cornflour and fried until crispy is really delicious and keeps this gluten-free alongside tamari instead of soy sauce.

Ingredients:

- 2 cups of basmati or other long-grain rice, cooked and cooled
- 1 onion, finely diced
- 5 medium mushrooms, thinly sliced

- 1 green pepper diced
- 1 cup of frozen edamame beans or garden peas
- Protein source such as soya chicken-style pieces, mince or tofu
- 1 heaped tsp of garlic-ginger paste
- ½ cup of soy sauce
- 1 tbsp of mirin
- 1 tsp of rice wine vinegar
- 1 tsp of agave or maple syrup
- 1 tsp of toasted sesame oil
- 1 tbsp of sesame seeds
- 4 spring onions, thinly sliced
- Oil for frying

Method:

1. Cook the rice as per my easy white rice recipe (in 'Sides and Salads'), and set aside for as long as possible, to avoid it being soggy instead of nice and chewy. Overnight in the fridge is best, but I often cook mine earlier in the daytime and fry it in the evening.
2. In a small bowl, whisk together the soy sauce, mirin, rice vinegar and syrup. Taste to make sure it's not too sweet or sharp, and adjust to your taste.
3. Heat a splash of oil in a wok and heat over a high flame. If you don't have a wok, just use a large frying pan. Once hot, add the onion, mushroom and pepper. You can also add your protein source at this point. Keep stirring or tossing over a high heat for 2–3 minutes. Once the vegetables and soya pieces or tofu are browning, add the garlic-ginger paste and keep stir-frying for another 30–60 seconds.

4. Add the rice to the pan and continue stir frying. If the rice is sticking very easily, add a small splash of oil. Fry for around 7 or 8 minutes, until the rice starts to colour slightly.

5. Use a wooden spoon or spatula to move all the rice into the centre of the wok, and pour your sauce down the edges of the pan so it caramelises just a little before it hits the rice. Then stir to combine it well, and cook for another 1–2 minutes before adding the edamame beans/peas. Keep cooking for another couple of minutes, until they are cooked.

6. Before removing the fried rice from the heat, drizzle it with sesame oil. Stir well and serve into 4 bowls, topping them with the sesame seeds and sliced spring onions.

Smoky Pepper and Tofu Stew with Buttery Bulgur Wheat

This serves 4 people, and is a fairly simple, easy dish to make, putting it firmly on my list of go-to mid-week staples. To make this gluten-free, use a suitable stock, use cornflour in place of plain flour, and a bulgur wheat alternative, like buckwheat or brown rice.

Ingredients:

- 3 sweet peppers, thickly sliced – I like a combination of red, orange and yellow
- 1 large onion, sliced
- 1 pack of extra-firm tofu, either smoked or regular, cut into 1cm cubes
- 1 tbsp of smoked paprika
- 1 tsp of ground cumin
- 1 tbsp of plain flour
- 2 cloves of garlic, finely chopped
- 400ml of vegan stock
- 1 tbsp of tomato puree
- 1 tin of cannellini beans (or any other white beans of your choice)
- Oil for cooking
- 1 cup of bulgur wheat

- 1 stock cube
- Salt and white pepper to season
- 2 heaped tbsp of vegan butter
- 4 tbsp of fresh parsley, finely chopped

Method:

1. Heat a splash of oil in a large frying pan, and once hot, add the onions. Fry for a few minutes until softened.
2. Add the sliced peppers to the pan with the garlic, and fry for 2–3 minutes until the smell of garlic is released. Don't let the garlic burn.
3. Add the paprika to the pan and fry for another 1–2 minutes. Pop a splash of stock into the pan and deglaze. Pour the rest of the stock in with the beans and cubed tofu. Bring it to the boil, then reduce to a simmer, pop a lid on and cook it for 30 minutes.
4. While the stew is simmering away, cook the bulgur wheat. Place it into a saucepan with 2 cups of boiling water. Crumble in the stock cube, stir well, and cover. Bring it to a boil, then simmer on a low heat for 10 minutes. Once the time is up, keep it covered for another 5–10 minutes, then take the lid off and stir through the butter and a pinch of white pepper to taste.
5. Once the casserole is cooked, remove it from the heat and season. Stir through the parsley, and serve it over the buttered bulgur wheat.

Sausage and White Bean Casserole with Dumplings

This recipe is another easy family dish, which is actually pretty flexible. You could use any sausage you fancy, and if you prefer you can keep the recipe entirely gluten-free by leaving the dumplings out, and choosing a suitable sausage and stock . I should also add that you could replace the sausages with any other protein source – but then I guess it wouldn't be a sausage casserole!

As for the beans, you could use any combination of white beans. I specify *white* beans, because I love the calcium content that comes in this great, fibre-filled dish. I've used butter beans and cannellini, but feel free to mix it up!

This recipe serves 4 with generous servings.

Ingredients:

(For the casserole)

- 8 vegan sausages
- 1 large onion, sliced
- 1 large carrot, sliced
- 1 large stick of celery
- 2 garlic cloves, finely chopped
- 2 tins of white beans, drained and rinsed
- 1 tbsp of Dijon or English mustard

- 750mls of vegan chicken-style stock
- 1 sprig of thyme
- 2 bay leaves
- A generous pinch of white pepper
- Oil for frying
- Salt to taste

(For the dumplings)

- 1 cup of plain flour
- 1 tsp of baking powder
- ¼ cup of vegan butter
- ½ cup of plant milk
- ½ tsp of dried sage
- Pinch of salt

Method:

1. In a shallow casserole dish, heat a splash of oil over a medium flame, then add the sausages and fry just until they've browned all over. Remove them from the pan with kitchen tongs, and place on a plate covered with a clean absorbent towel to remove any excess oil.
2. Add the onion, carrot and celery to the pan and fry for a few minutes over a medium heat until softened, then add the garlic and thyme, and continue cooking for another minute or two.
3. Add the beans, stock, mustard, and bay leaves. Bring the casserole to a boil, then reduce to a simmer, and cook with the lid on for 30 minutes.

4. While the casserole is simmering away, make the dumplings. Add the flour, sage, and baking powder to a large mixing bowl and stir together. Cut in the vegan butter to make a crumbly mixture. I do this with a fork by kind of 'mashing' the flour and fat together. Then slowly stir in the milk until you've got a rough, lumpy batter. Let it sit until you're ready to use it.

5. Check the casserole, and stir from time to time, to make sure nothing is sticking or burning. When the 30 minutes are up, season to taste, then add the sausages, spacing them out to keep room for the dumplings. Dollop the dumpling batter into these spaces to make 'dumpling islands' that are half submerged. There should be roughly 8 small dumplings. Add more stock if the casserole is looking dry. The dumplings will absorb a fair bit of liquid. Replace the lid and cook on low for 15 minutes.

6. This should be eaten immediately, but if you are planning on waiting to eat it, then don't add the dumpling batter until 15 minutes before serving, when you can cook them freshly, to avoid them drying out, and reheat the casserole at the same time.

I really like this with mustard mash, but it would also work with quinoa, rice or roast potatoes.

Puy Lentil Cottage Pie

I love this dish. Despite my passion for world foods, I also love a cosy British dish sometimes, and I adore finding ways to make these family favourites vegan. I've made a thousand versions of cottage pie, with various fillings and toppings, but my all-time favourite is this one, with earthy Puy lentils, and a gorgeous, rich miso mash on top. You can swap other veggies into the lentil mix, and replace the mince with extra lentils, or perhaps chopped mushrooms. I think the combination of flavours I've used here really is delicious, though. With the right stock and gravy granules, this is another recipe which can easily be made gluten-free.

This pie serves 4 people, and goes very well with tangy brown sauce and a side of pickles or sauerkraut.

Ingredients:

- 2 large baking potatoes
- 1 butternut squash
- 1 onion, finely chopped
- 1 large carrot, finely chopped
- 2 sticks of celery, finely chopped
- 2 garlic cloves, finely chopped
- 1 pack of refrigerated vegan mince
- 1 cup of Puy lentils
- 2 bay leaves
- 1 heaped tsp of dried sage

- 1 heaped tsp of dried rosemary
- 1 small sprig of fresh thyme
- 750mls of stock
- 50g of vegan butter
- 1 tbsp of miso paste
- 3 tbsp of vegan gravy granules
- Oil for frying

Method:

1. Heat the oven to 200C. Cut the squash into large pieces and transfer to a couple of baking trays, toss in oil and cook in the middle of the oven for 45 minutes. Turn once during cooking.
2. Peel and chop the potatoes into 1cm pieces. Boil a pan of water and add the potatoes. Cook until soft and easy to break when poked with a fork.
3. Rinse and drain the lentils and place them into a saucepan. Cover them with water, bring to a boil, and cook for 20 minutes.
4. Heat a splash of oil in a large pan or casserole dish. Add the onions, celery and carrot and sauté until softened.
5. Add the mince to the pan, break it up with a fork, and cook until browned. Add the herbs, bay leaf and garlic, and fry for a further 2 minutes.
6. Add the lentils and stock to the pan with the mince and combine well. Bring to the boil, then reduce and simmer for half an hour.
7. In a microwaveable jug or bowl, dissolve the miso paste in a splash of boiled water, then add the butter. Microwave for 30

seconds, stir, and repeat for another 30 seconds if the butter hasn't fully melted.

8. Transfer the boiled potatoes to a large mixing bowl. Remove the skin from the butternut squash and put this in the bowl too. Add the miso butter mix to the bowl, and mash well.

9. Take the lid off the mince and lentils, add 3 heaped table-spoons of gravy and stir well.

10. Transfer the lentil and mince mix to a large oven dish and make sure it's evenly distributed through the whole bowl. Spoon the mash on top, and gently spread it out with the back of a spoon. Use a fork to make lines up and down the length of the pie for extra crunchiness, or if you're feeling re-ally fancy, blend the mash to a puree and pipe onto the pie.

11. Place the pie into the hot oven, and cook on the middle shelf for 30 minutes.

Mushroom Stroganoff

This creamy, vegan version of an old favourite serves 4 people, and is great with various choices of side dishes. I particularly like it with orzo pasta and a salad, but it also works with rice or mashed potato. It takes less than half an hour to cook, making a good mid-week staple after a busy day. It's gluten-free, too.

Ingredients:

- 500g mushrooms – I like to use a combination of white and chestnut, button and baby button, sliced and halved/quartered for texture
- 3 echalion shallots, halved then finely sliced
- A large bunch of parsley, roughly chopped, around 25g
- 250ml of vegan cream – soya or oat is fine
- 1 tbsp of paprika
- 1 tbsp of Dijon mustard – you can add extra if you particularly like the mustard flavour, or if your mustard is very mild
- 30ml of brandy
- 2 tbsp of oil for frying

Method:

1. Heat the oil in a heavy pan over a medium heat.
2. Add the shallots and cook for a few minutes until they are soft, and starting to brown.

3. Add the mushrooms and a splash more oil if it is all quickly absorbed or the mushrooms stick.
4. Once the mushrooms have softened add half of the parsley and the paprika, and continue frying for 3–4 minutes, stirring so the mushrooms don't stick.
5. Add the brandy to the pan and allow the alcohol to cook off for a few minutes before adding the mustard and simmering for a couple more minutes.
6. Add the soya cream and stir well so that all of the ingredients are combined, and simmer for 5–10 minutes
7. Add the rest of the parsley just before serving.

Giant Samosa Pie

There's not a lot to say about this one; it's like a samosa, but giant! What's not to love? I have made this with both filo and puff pastry, and whilst both were great, I love crisp filo wrapped around the soft potatoes. This version contains vegan mince, used as a keema, but I've also made it without and it was equally lovely. Also feel free to mix up your veggies to your liking, and use variations on mince that work for your needs. If you have a gluten-free diet, use a puff pastry which is made without.

This pie will serve a family of 4 with side dishes.

Ingredients:

- 3 large potatoes, peeled and cut into 0.5–1cm cubes
- 2 large carrots, peeled and cut into 0.5cm cubes
- 1 medium onion, finely chopped
- 2 cloves of garlic, finely chopped
- 2 tsp of minced ginger
- 1 cup of frozen peas
- ½ cup of fresh coriander, big stalks removed and the rest roughly chopped
- 1 pack of vegan mince
- 1 tsp of fennel seeds
- 1 tsp of mustard seeds
- 1 tsp of cumin seeds

- 1 tsp of turmeric
- 1 tsp of ground coriander
- 1 tsp of ground cumin
- 2 tsp of garam masala
- 1 pack of filo pastry
- Oil for cooking
- Olive oil for brushing the pastry

Method:

1. Heat the oven to 200°C and fill a saucepan with boiling water, placing it over a high flame to get it to a boil. Add your cubed potatoes and boil them for 5 minutes. They will still be a bit firm, but don't worry. They only need to be parboiled at this point.
2. In a large sauté pan or shallow casserole dish, heat a generous splash of oil. Once it is hot, tip in your vegan mince, and use a wooden spoon to break it all up. Fry until it is crispy in places, stirring frequently.
3. Use a slotted spoon to remove the mince from the pan, and leave it to one side in a bowl. Rinse the pan and dry well.
4. Add another splash of oil to the pan, and place it over a medium heat. Once it's hot, tip in your mustard, fennel and cumin seeds, and fry until they start to pop.
5. Add the onion and carrot to the hot oil and sauté for around 5 minutes until they start to soften.
6. Add the ginger and garlic to the pan and cook for another minute before adding the ground spices. Cook for 1 minute to release the aroma of the spices, then tip in the potatoes. Fry

for 3–4 minutes, then add 1 cup of water. Cover and simmer for 5 minutes.

7. Remove the lid, stir well, and add the peas to the pan. If the liquid has all been absorbed, add another cup of water. Replace the lid and simmer gently for another 5 minutes.

8. Take the pan off the heat, remove the lid, and stir through the chopped fresh coriander and the fried mince and leave it to cool, whilst removing your pastry from the fridge, and let it come to room temperature for a few minutes.

9. Carefully open the pastry, making sure not to break the sheets. The occasional break won't matter too much, but you don't want too many tears. Pour a little olive oil into a small bowl, then use a pastry brush to grease the pie dish.

10. Take one sheet of the pastry and place it in the oven dish, tucking it into the corners. Brush this layer with olive oil, and then place another sheet on top. Turn the second sheet 90 degrees so that the longer side of the sheet runs in the opposite direction to the first; for example, the first sheet could be longest running vertically, then the second longest from side to side. Repeat the process with the third sheet, placing it in the same direction as the first.

11. Tip the veggies and mince into the dish, and use the back of a wooden spoon or spatula to press it down firmly into all edges and corners. Pull the long edges of the sheets of filo over the top of the contents, allowing them to wrinkle a bit.

12. Use the remaining sheets by wrinkling them up into scrunchy little bundles and placing them on top of the pie, covering the whole surface. Use the pastry brush to put a light coating of olive oil over the whole thing.

13. Place the pie in the centre of the heated oven and cook for 25 minutes. If the pastry isn't crisp and brown at this point, pop it back in for another 5 minutes.

It goes beautifully with buttered cabbage with fennel seeds (see page 320) and buttered bulgur wheat.

Green Lentil and Soya Mince Lasagne

This recipe will serve 4–6 people and takes a little time and love to make, but it's all worth it when you're sat around the family dinner table tucking in to this comfort food classic.

Ingredients:

(For the bolognese)

- 1 onion, finely chopped
- 2 celery sticks, finely sliced
- 1 large carrot, finely chopped
- 2 cloves of garlic, finely chopped
- ½ tsp of dried oregano
- ½ tsp of dried basil
- 1 tbsp of red wine vinegar
- 4 large, ripe tomatoes, roughly chopped or 2 tins of chopped tomatoes
- 2 tbsp of tomato puree
- 1 tsp of sugar
- 500ml of vegetable stock
- 1 tin of cooked green lentils
- 1 cup of dried soya mince, rehydrated
- 1 tsp of yeast extract
- 1 tbsp of olive oil

(For the béchamel sauce)

- 1½ tbsp of vegan butter
- ¼ cup of plain flour
- 300ml of plant milk
- 1 pinch of nutmeg
- 1 pinch of salt

(To make the lasagne)

- 1 pack of egg-free lasagne sheets
- A handful of grated vegan cheese
- 1 tablespoon of nutritional yeast (optional)

Method:

Heat the oven to 200°C.

(For the bolognese)

1. Heat the olive oil over a medium heat in a large sauté or saucepan.
2. Add the onion, celery, carrot, garlic, oregano and basil, and cook for 3–4 minutes until softened.
3. Add the red wine vinegar and simmer for 2 minutes.
4. Add the chopped tomatoes to the pan and cook for a further 3–4 minutes.
5. Sprinkle the sugar over the contents of the pan, then add the stock, tomato puree, yeast extract. Stir well and leave to simmer for 5–10 minutes.

6. Add the lentils, and allow to simmer for another 15 minutes. For a fuller flavour, you can let this simmer for a lot longer, but make sure you don't let it dry out.

(For the béchamel sauce)

1. Melt the butter over a gentle heat.
2. When melted, add the flour, mixing well to form a paste. Continue stirring for a minute or two to cook the flour. The mixture should change colour to a darker yellow.
3. Over a low heat, taking it off from time to time if it's getting too hot, add the milk a splash at a time, mixing well to avoid forming lumps.
4. Once all the milk has been added, keep stirring and simmer for another 2 minutes, adding further splashes of milk if the sauce is too thick.
5. Take the sauce off the heat and stir through the nutmeg and salt.

(Building your lasagne)

1. Use a large oven dish which will fit a lasagne for 4–6 people. Mine is 18 x 28cm. Cover the bottom of the dish with lasagne sheets – depending on the shape and size of your dish, you might have to break some of the sheets. If you do this, make sure there are no gaps between the pieces of pasta.
2. Spoon some bolognese sauce over the layer of lasagne; it's up to you how thick you want your layers to be.
3. Cover this layer of sauce with lasagne sheets, and continue alternating between pasta and sauce until you have no sauce left. As my dish is quite long, I only usually have 2 or 3 layers. If

your dish is deeper but smaller, you might get 4 or 5 layers. Make sure you finish with a layer of pasta on top.

4. Pour the béchamel over the top of the lasagne, making sure it is all covered with sauce, and cook in the centre of the oven for 20 minutes.

5. Remove the lasagne from the oven, and sprinkle over your vegan cheese. You can also add a sprinkle of nutritional yeast flakes for extra flavour and a dose of vitamin B12.

6. Cook for a further 10 minutes.

Slice the lasagne into 4 or 6 portions (depending on your appetite), and serve with a fresh, green salad tossed in olive oil and balsamic vinegar.

Parippu

(Sri Lankan Lentil Curry)

I first learned how to make this dish when I was trying to impress my partner's family who hail from Sri Lanka. I've since 'veganised' the dish and have made it for them with great feedback. It's loaded with iron-rich lentils and, surprisingly, the coconut milk also has a good iron content. This recipe serves 4 people as a light meal or with other curries, but if you are eating it as a main course with just rice and salad, it'll be good for 2 people. This is a naturally gluten-free recipe without any adjustments being made.

This dish is cooked in 2 parts but it's really easy, and you can take a portion for babies and toddlers out of the pan before you temper it, as this makes it a little spicy.

Ingredients:

(For the lentil curry)

- 1 cup of red split lentils
- 1 cinammon stick
- 6 dried red chilli peppers
- ½ red onion, finely chopped
- 1 medium to large tomato, roughly chopped

- 1 tsp of turmeric
- 1 cup of water
- 2 cups of coconut milk

(To temper)

- 1 tsp of mustard seeds – I use black mustard seeds
- 1 tsp of chopped ginger
- 1 tsp of chopped garlic
- ½ tsp of dried chilli flakes
- 10 dried curry leaves
- 1 tbsp of oil or vegan butter

Method:

1. Add the lentils, cinnamon, whole dried chilli peppers, onion, tomato, turmeric, water and coconut milk to a saucepan. Bring the mix to the boil, then reduce to a simmer, stirring occasionally to ensure the lentils aren't sticking to the bottom of the pan. Cook for around 15 minutes, adding a splash of water if the lentils become dry before they have softened.
2. Whilst the lentils are cooking, put the oil into a small saucepan, and place over a moderate heat. Once the oil is hot, add the mustard seeds and heat until they begin to pop.
3. Then add the ginger, curry leaves and chilli flakes and fry for 2–3 minutes.
4. Turn the heat down and add the garlic. This is added last so it doesn't burn. Fry for another 1–2 minutes.
5. Add the spice mix to the lentils, and stir through. If the lentils haven't softened, cook for another 5 minutes, or until the liq-

uid has absorbed. Don't forget to add a splash of water if the liquid has been absorbed and the lentils aren't soft enough.

6. Serve with rice and seeni sambol, or alongside any other Sri Lankan curries as a side dish. Parippu is also great to dunk crusty buttered bread into!

Love Heart Pie

(Chick'n, mushroom and sweetcorn pie)

Sometimes you find a vegan dish that's just so good, you wonder why anybody bothers making or eating an omnivore version. This pie is one of them. I just love the fact that pre-made pastries are generally vegan-friendly. It makes cooking what could be complicated dishes, like this, so easy. I use the excess pastry that comes away when I trim it to decorate the top of mine with a little love heart. That's why my eldest child has called this one Love Heart Pie, and the name just stuck.

As with most of my recipes, this one is flexible. You can replace the tofu with vegan chicken-style pieces if you like, or even throw in a few tins of white beans of different varieties. You can add other vegetables if you wish; peas might be nice, or even carrots, broccoli or chickpeas. The crux of this dish is the creamy dill and mustard sauce that wraps it all together.

Feel free to switch your pastry and flour to gluten-free versions, or if you want to keep it more whole-food based, you can top the pie filling with mashed or sliced potatoes.

This serves 6 with a side of vegetables.

Ingredients:

- 4 tbsp of vegan butter
- 4 tbsp of plain flour
- 400ml of plant milk
- 250ml of vegan stock – I like chicken style for this recipe
- 1 tbsp of finely chopped fresh dill, larger stalks removed
- 1 tbsp of Dijon mustard
- 2–4 shallots (depending on size), halved lengthwise and thinly sliced – a white or brown onion would be fine in place of this
- 250g of mushrooms, chopped – I like chestnut mushrooms, but most types would be fine, and depending on the size, you can slice, half, or quarter them
- 2 garlic cloves, finely chopped
- 450g of extra firm tofu cut into small cubes
- 1 small tin of sweetcorn, drained
- A 400g tin of cannellini beans – other white beans would also work
- Oil for cooking
- Salt and white pepper for seasoning
- 1 pack of ready-made, rolled puff pastry

Method:

1. Heat the oven to 200C and take the pastry out of the fridge.
2. We're going to start by making the sauce, which is based on a béchamel sauce. To do this, melt the butter in a saucepan over a low to medium heat. Add the flour and cook it for a few minutes, to make a roux. The colour will change a little, turning slightly darker, but make sure you don't burn it.

3. Mix the milk with the hot stock in a large jug, then add this gradually to the roux, 50–100ml at a time, stirring continuously to avoid lumps. Once all the milk and stock is added, pop in the dill and mustard, stir it well, and season with salt and white pepper to taste. Now is the time to add a bit more mustard if you fancy a bit more tang.

4. Bring the sauce to a boil for a moment, give it one final stir, then take the pan of the heat and cover it with a lid to avoid a skin forming on top.

5. If you have a shallow casserole dish that will go into the oven, use this. Otherwise use a deep sauté pan, add a splash of oil, and heat it over a medium flame. Add the shallots and sauté until softened and starting to brown. Next add the mushrooms and fry until they are softened and pretty much cooked. If they start sticking to the pan add another splash of oil. Add the garlic and cook for a further minute until the aroma of the garlic is released, then season and take off the heat.

6. Add the tofu cubes and sweetcorn to the dish, and stir it well to combine everything. Pour the sauce over the mushroom and chick'n mixture, and stir well. If you are using a casserole dish that will transfer to the oven, then scrape the sauce down off the edges. If you are going to use a pie tin, then transfer it now. Leave everything to cool down for 15 minutes or so.

7. Roll out your pastry on a floured surface, making sure to roll it big enough to fit over your dish. Transfer it onto your pie filling, tucking it into the edges, and cut off any excess. Use either a fork or a finger to pinch it against the pie dish all the way around. Put a couple of small holes in the top with a sharp knife, and decorate with any excess pastry if you wish.

8. Brush the pie top all over with a little plant milk, then pop it into the middle of the oven. I usually check it at 25 minutes as my oven isn't always reliable, but around 30 minutes, give or take 5 minutes either side usually does the job. If your pie is still looking a bit pale at 30 minutes, give it another 5.

9. Serve it with mashed or roasted potatoes and my buttered cabbage with fennel seeds for a cosy, hearty meal, or with a nice salad for a light lunch.

Chick'n and Pearl Barley Harissa Casserole

This delicious casserole has a lovely warmth from the harissa, with little bites of sweetness throughout from the apricots, and a hit of herby freshness with the coriander. It's all cooked in one large pot, which keeps things simple, too. To make this gluten free, you could replace the barley with brown rice, buckwheat or quinoa, but you will need to reduce your cooking time and liquid quantity appropriately.

This serves 4, with big, hearty portions.

Ingredients:

- 2 packs or 500g (ish) of vegan chicken pieces (soya, or seitan, or pea protein will do)
- 1 cup of pearl barley
- 4 tablespoons of rose harissa – adjust to preferred spiciness level
- 2 large carrots, thickly sliced – peel them if you prefer, but I keep the skins on
- 1 large onion, thinly sliced
- 1 tin of chickpeas, drained
- A handful of dried apricots, roughly chopped – these can be replaced with jumbo raisins or chopped dates, either of which are also tasty and nutritious

- A handful of fresh coriander, chopped – if you are one of those people that really doesn't like the taste of coriander, you can replace this with parsley
- 750mls of vegan stock – I use vegan chicken-style stock, but vegetable will also work well
- ¼ cup of tahini
- 1 tbsp of lemon juice
- 1 tsp of maple syrup
- Oil for cooking

Method:

1. Heat a splash of oil in a large sauté or frying pan, and add the onion and gently fry over a low heat. Once softened, add the chick'n pieces and carrots and fry for a further 5 minutes.
2. Add the harissa and barley to the pan and stir well to cover everything in the harissa, and cook for a few minutes, stirring to avoid anything sticking.
3. Put the stock and chickpeas into the pan, bring to the boil, then reduce to a simmer and cook for 30 minutes with a lid on.
4. Stir the contents of the pan well, and check how wet everything is. Add more stock if necessary, then add the apricots, re-cover, and cook for a further 15–20 minutes. Make sure the pan doesn't turn dry and burn. Add a splash of stock where required.
5. While the casserole is cooking, make your tahini sauce. Put the tahini, lemon juice and maple syrup into a small bowl, and whisk it together. If it is stiff, add a splash of warm water to loosen.

6. Take the pan off the heat, and stir through the coriander. Serve drizzled with the tahini dressing, alongside a salad and flatbreads.

B ibimbap

It only took me about 6 hours in Korea to discover what was going to become one of my favourite dishes, and I've been eating it ever since. We'd arrived in Seoul for the start of a 2-month trip around Korea and China, and after dropping our bags at the hostel, we were hungry and on the search for something delectable. I saw a picture of bibimbap, checked it was vegetarian (I wasn't yet vegan), and sat down to wait for my order. A delicious pile of veggies and rice came topped with an egg. On the side was a little dish of hot red sauce – gochujang sauce.

We must have looked like we didn't know where to start! A lovely, elderly lady reminded me very much of my late nanna when she came over to our table, curtly took the spoon from my hand, and began to roughly chop and mix all the ingredients in my bowl, adding the sauce, and mixing some more. I'm so glad she did, as I would have hesitantly picked at all of the tasty vegetables, not realising it's meant to be a beautiful, spicy mess.

Silken tofu replaces the egg in my version, and I use soya mince where some would add meat. If you're in a pinch for time, use pouches of microwave rice, and just stir fry all the vegetables together and pile them on top. You'll reduce your cooking time considerably, and you'll still enjoy a comforting, nutritious meal. Crumbled or grated tofu also work in place of soya mince.

This serves 4 people. Make sure to get stuck in, mix it all up, and enjoy.

Ingredients:

- 2 cups of white rice, cooked as per instructions
- Roughly 250g, or around 2 trays of shiitake mushrooms, roughly sliced
- 3 large carrots, cut into batons (It's up to you if you peel them, I don't.)
- 1 large bag of spinach, around 300g
- 400g of soya mince – the refrigerated or frozen type works best for this, rather than dried soya mince
- 1 pack of extra-firm silken tofu – this must be silken tofu for its soft texture
- 6 tbsp of gochujang paste
- 2 tsp of rice wine vinegar
- 1 tbsp of mirin
- 100mls of soy sauce
- 2 tbsp of maple or agave syrup
- Sesame seeds – I like toasted black sesame seeds
- 1 tbsp of toasted sesame oil
- Oil for frying

Method:

1. Cook your rice as per my white rice instructions (see p.316).
2. Heat a splash of oil in a large frying pan or wok and stir fry the carrot batons for a few minutes, but stopping before they soften too much. Remove them from the heat and place them in a bowl lined with absorbent paper towel. Repeat this step with the mushrooms.

3. Next add a splash of sesame oil to the pan and wilt the spinach. Again, remove from the pan to a bowl, then rinse the pan out, before putting it back on the heat and adding a splash of vegetable oil. Fry the soya mince until it starts to crisp, then pour in 1 tbsp of the soy sauce and stir well. Remove it from the heat.

4. In a small bowl, mix the gochujang, the remaining soy sauce, vinegar, mirin and syrup. Combine well and make sure there are no lumps, then keep it to one side to use shortly.

5. Carefully slice the tofu into eight slices, being careful not to break it. It is rather delicate (and wobbly!), so just take your time.

6. It's time to build your bibimbap. Split the rice into four bowls. Top with the vegetables and soya mince. To keep it traditional keep each ingredient in its own little pile. Next place two slices of tofu on top of the rice and vegetables, before drizzling with the gochujang sauce. Sprinkle with sesame seeds and admire the lovely colours before it gets mixed up and devoured!

'Duck' and Udon Noodles in a Curried Broth

This hearty noodle soup was inspired by a favourite dish of mine from a well-known Pan-Asian restaurant that does vegan food particularly well. That one contains crispy-coated silken tofu, but I've never been very good at coating pieces of delicate silken tofu! Instead I like to use tinned 'mock-duck', the wonderful braised seitan that you can buy from East Asian supermarkets, but you could use any protein source you like, or even leave these out and just use extra chopped veggies.

This recipe serves 4, and is quite a satisfying meal due to the full-fat coconut milk, alongside whichever protein source you opt for, and the lovely chewy noodles. To make this gluten free, use a suitable stock cube, and replace the udon with rice noodles or authentic soba noodles which shouldn't contain any gluten.

Ingredients:

- 1 medium onion, thinly sliced
- 4 cloves of garlic
- 2 tbsp of minced ginger
- 4 tbsp of mild curry powder
- 2 tins of full fat coconut milk
- 1 litre of stock (vegan chicken-style)
- 4 medium carrots, cut into batons
- 1 pack of chestnut mushrooms
- 1 pack of washed baby spinach

- 1 cup of sweetcorn
- 4 packs of ready-made udon noodles
- 1 tin of mock-duck or any meat replacement which cooks to crispy when fried
- Oil for cooking

Method:

1. Heat a splash of oil in a saucepan, then add the onion, frying over a medium heat for 2 minutes.
2. Add the garlic and ginger and cook for another 3 minutes, being careful not to burn the garlic.
3. Add the curry powder and cook for a further 1 minute, stirring frequently.
4. Add the stock and coconut milk, bring them to a boil, then reduce the heat and simmer whilst cooking the other components.
5. Heat a splash of oil in a frying pan then add carrots and cook for 2 minutes. Then add mushrooms and fry until they are cooked through. Remove the vegetables from the pan to a plate lined with a clean absorbant towel to remove excess oil.
6. Add the pieces of mock duck to the hot pan and fry them until crispy. Once ready, remove them from the pan to the paper-lined plate to remove excess oil.
7. Stir the spinach through broth to wilt it and add the noodles. Simmer for 2 minutes until the noodles feel soft.
8. Divide noodle into 2 bowls, ladle on the broth and top it all with the veggies. Finish with the crispy mock duck.

Sides and Salads

Nanna's Crispy Roast Potatoes

My nanna was in no way vegan, but her very non-vegan roast dinners included the most delicious potatoes known to humans. Well, to our family, at least. And my mum and dad have been making them the same way ever since, so it's no surprise, really, that I make my potatoes the exact same way. And that they get the same positive response that Nanna's did.

When I sat down to write this recipe out, I put a note next to the title saying *'measure potato weight, oil mls and flour weight'*, because in the 25 years I've been making this side dish, I've never once done any of these things. I told you I'm a relaxed cook, didn't I? But I then decided, you know what? I'm going to describe just how I cook it, and you should be able to get the same result. So, here goes.

This should make enough roast potatoes for 3–4 people.

Ingredients:

- Lots of potatoes, maybe around 1–2kg, or just over half of a large bag
- Plain flour – maybe half to one cup, and this can be subbed for cornflour if you are gluten free

- Oil, lots, see below. We use rapeseed oil for this, but I think olive oil or sunflower would also work
- Salt and black pepper to season

Method:

1. Heat your oven to 190°C and pour your oil of choice into a large roasting dish to a depth of around 1cm. Once the oven comes to temperature, pop the dish into the middle of the oven.
2. Boil a kettle of water and peel your potatoes. Cut them into a mixture of shapes and sizes. I cut small potatoes in half, and larger ones into 4 or 6 pieces.
3. Pop your boiled water into a large saucepan and bring to the boil again over a high heat. Put the potatoes in once the water is boiling, and keep over a high heat until the water is bubbling again.
4. Turn the heat down and simmer the potatoes until they are soft enough to break with a fork.
5. Remove them from the heat and drain with a colander. Once every drop of water has drained off, return them to the pan. Pour your flour over and toss the pan up and down until the flour has coated the potatoes. You can season them now, too if you want to use salt.
6. Carefully remove the roasting dish from the oven, and keeping your body and face away, tip the pan of potatoes away from you into the hot oil. Wear oven gloves to avoid oil splashes on your hands, too. Turn the potatoes, making sure that they all get a coating of hot oil. If the oil was hot enough you should hear a big sizzle when you first tip the potatoes in, then smaller sizzles as you turn them and the oil cools a bit.

7. Return the roasting dish to the oven and cook for 30 minutes.

8. Remove the potatoes from the oven and turn them all. Some might be a little stuck on the bottom, but if you carefully try to lift away even the stuck bit, you should get some nice crispy edges coming away.

9. Put the dish back in the oven for around 15 minutes. By then the potatoes should be browned and crispy, but if you need a bit longer, pop them back in, checking at 15 minute intervals.

10. Place the potatoes on clean kitchen towel to remove oil prior to serving with either a hearty roast dinner, or any other main of your choice.

Easy White Rice Recipe

At the risk of being accused of trying to tell you something far too straight-forward (I'm remembering a celebrity chef who was laughed at for telling people how to boil an egg in one of her books), I think cooking rice is something that should be so easy, but that you can get very wrong. There are different methods all over the internet, and I've found that many of them are inconsistent in their results for a nice fluffy rice.

So here's how I cook mine. One complication is that when I changed my saucepan set, I found that the quantity of water I needed changed. I suggest that if you're following my method, start with the quantities I suggest, and if the end result is a bit dry, add an extra quarter cup of water next time. If it's too wet, then use a quarter cup less on your next attempt.

This makes enough for 2 people for a large portion.

Ingredients:

- 1 cup of white long-grain rice (we use basmati)

Method:

1. In the saucepan you are going to use, wash the rice with cold water, using your hand to swirl it around, tipping the water out, and repeating this three times.
2. After the final wash and rinse, use a strainer to drain the rice, and pop it back into the pan.
3. Boil a kettle, then add 1.5 cups of boiled water to the rice, stir, cover and bring to a boil. Once it's bubbling, reduce the heat to a very gentle simmer and allow it to cook for 8 minutes.
4. When your cooking time is up, turn off the heat, but don't remove the lid. Set the time again for 5 minutes, to allow the rice to steam.
5. After 5 minutes, remove the lid and use a wooden spoon or chopstick to fluff the rice up. It's ready to eat.

Warm Quinoa and Butternut Squash Salad

This is such a simple dish to make, but it's really tasty and full of goodness. During the summer months I like to keep a big dish of this in the fridge to go with other salads for nights when it is too warm to cook or eat hot food. Quinoa is a fantastic source of protein and butternut squash is full of fibre and vitamin C, and goes really well with quinoa when it's roasted. This is gluten-free with the right vegetable stock.

Serves 4 as a main dish, more if serving with other salads.

Ingredients:

- 1 medium-sized butternut squash
- 1 cup of quinoa
- 500mls of vegetable stock
- 1 heaped cup of rocket, rinsed
- 3 tbsp of cold-pressed rapeseed oil or extra virgin olive oil
- 1 tsp of red chilli flakes
- Salt and pepper to taste

Method:

1. Heat oven to 180°C and cut the squash into small wedges of around 1 inch long. I like to leave the skin on, but feel free to peel it if this isn't for you. You can also remove the skin from the squash after it has been cooked.

2. Pour the oil into a large roasting tin, then throw in the pieces of squash. Sprinkle over the chilli flakes, toss the pieces so they are all covered in oil and chilli flakes, and put into the middle of the oven for 30 minutes.

3. In a saucepan, add the quinoa to the vegetable stock and bring it to the boil. Turn down the heat and allow it to simmer for 10–15 minutes, checking every now and then that it hasn't boiled dry. Just add another splash of stock or water if it does. You'll be able to see a white ring on the grains of quinoa when it is cooked, and it should still have a little bite.

4. Once the butternut squash has roasted for 30 minutes, take it out of the oven and check that the pieces are all soft. Season it to your preference.

5. Leave the squash to cool down, and transfer the cooked quinoa to a mixing bowl, adding the squash once it has cooled, including the oil and juices from the roasting tin.

6. Stir the rocket through and serve warm.

Buttered Cabbage with Fennel Seeds

This is a delicious side dish, but in all honesty I could eat a great big bowl of it. It goes fantastically with the Chick'n, Mushroom and Sweetcorn Pie, but you could even serve it with Parippu or any other curry.

Ingredients:

- Half of a sweetheart or large savoy cabbage
- 3 tbsp of vegan butter
- 1 heaped tbsp of fennel seeds
- Salt and black pepper to taste

Method:

1. Using a large sharp knife, half the cabbage again, remove the core, and slice thinly.
2. Use a large sauté pan to heat the butter over a medium heat.
3. Add the fennel seeds and allow them to sizzle for 1–2 minutes.
4. Add the cabbage and stir fry for 5 minutes or so until the cabbage has softened and is coated in butter. Season and serve.

Herby Bulgur Wheat Salad

In our family, I'm known for my salads, and I always joke that no-body makes salad like a vegan. We tend to have a few on rotation in the fridge over the summer, and this one is a favourite, full of fibre and protein. It's great on its own for a nutritious lunch to take to work, or alongside lots of other dishes for a leisurely summer lunch in the garden. You could even serve it with something hot, like a casserole, for a main course. The base of bulgur wheat means it's not naturally gluten-free, but you could replace this with another suitable grain.

This should be enough for 3 or 4 people as a light lunch, or more if served with other salads or as a side dish.

Ingredients:

- 1 cup of bulgur wheat
- 500mls of stock – I like vegan chicken-style for this dish
- 4 spring onions
- Half a punnet of cherry tomatoes
- 1 tin of black beans, drained and rinsed
- 1 cup of sweetcorn
- Juice of half a lemon
- A small bunch of parsley, finely chopped
- 2 tbsp of extra virgin olive oil
- Rose harissa to serve

Method:

1. Place the bulgur wheat in a pan with the stock. Bring to the boil, then turn the heat down and simmer for around 10 minutes. Take the pan off the heat, but keep the lid on for another 5 minutes to allow the wheat to keep steaming.
2. Whilst the bulgur wheat is cooking, finely slice your spring onions, and cut the tomatoes into quarters. Finely chop the parsley leaves, and discard the stalks.
3. Once the bulgur wheat has cooked, leave it to cool before placing it in a large mixing bowl.
4. Add the chopped veg and herbs to the bowl and mix well. Add the lemon juice and olive oil, and mix well to combine.
5. When you are ready to serve, pop a teaspoon (or more if you prefer) of harissa over each portion.

Rice and Peas

This is one of those dishes that I've changed and perfected over the years to one that is super easy to make, with maximum flavour. It's our go-to quick evening meal after a day at work, served with something wonderfully warm and spicy like jerk or curry. I always think that a tangy slaw finishes it off nicely, too.

This serves 3–4 depending on what you're eating it with.

Ingredients:

- 1 cup of basmati rice, rinsed and drained
- 1 tin of coconut milk
- 1 sprig of fresh thyme
- 3 spring onions, thinly sliced
- 1 tsp of ground allspice
- 1 tin of kidney beans in water (don't drain these)
- Salt, to taste

Method:

1. Place all of the ingredients into a saucepan, including the water the beans came in, stir well, cover and place over the heat.

2. Bring to a boil, then reduce to a simmer and cook for 10 minutes.

3. Turn the heat off, but keep the lid on for another 2–3 minutes. Season and serve.

Simple Salad Dressing

A good salad dressing can make a few leaves into something really special. I like to make this one in a glass jar with a screw-on lid, so the ingredients can be shaken together and the dressing stored leaving no dishes to wash!

Ingredients:

- ½ cup of cold pressed rapeseed oil
- 2 tbsp of sherry vinegar
- 1 tsp of fresh thyme, chopped
- 1 tbsp of agave syrup
- 1 tsp of dijon mustard
- Salt, to taste

Method:

1. Place all of the above ingredients into a jar, screw on the lid, and shake, shake, shake. When the oil, mustard and vinegar have mixed well and emulsified, it's ready to use, or to pop into the fridge for later. Just don't forget to give it another shake when you're ready to use it.

Puddings

Rich and Creamy Chocolate Pudding

I don't have a huge repertoire of desserts, but this is one that gets made over and over, because it is just so luscious. This pudding has the bonus of the nutrient profile of tofu, meaning it's rich in calcium, fibre and protein. You'd never know that when you're tucking in, of course.

This recipe serves four, with small portions, as it is very rich.

Ingredients:

- 1 carton of extra firm silken tofu
- 100g of dark chocolate
- 1 tbsp of cocoa powder or cacao
- ½ tbsp of date syrup (this can be left out, increased for extra sweetness, or replaced with another syrup of your preference)
- 1tsp of vanilla extract
- 1 tbsp of chopped, roasted hazelnuts (you can toast chopped hazelnuts on a dry frying pan, or buy them ready roasted)

Method:

1. Break your chocolate into cubes, and place them in a microwaveable bowl. Put them into the microwave on full power for 1 minute. Give them a stir, and if the chocolate hasn't all melted when you've mixed it well, pop it in for another 20 seconds. Keep doing this until it's all melted.
2. Open the carton of tofu, and carefully drain any liquid out. Pop the block of tofu into your food processor or blender with the melted chocolate, cocoa powder, vanilla extract and date syrup.
3. Whizz it up for 30–60 seconds, then check the flavour. If you think it needs more cocoa for chocolatiness, or syrup for sweetness, the pop some in. Blend the mixture again for another 30–60 seconds.
4. Transfer it into two dessert dishes, and sprinkle the chopped nuts between the two.
5. Refrigerate for at least two hours, then enjoy. Leaving it overnight does ensure it's really thick and set.

Final Thoughts

A fter reading this book, I hope it's clear that not only are there so many reasons to live vegan, but that they are all so very interconnected. Connections are important, and often what our modern lives are lacking. Re-finding these, and working out how we are connected with those around us, our planet and its non-human inhabitants, and even our own mind, body, and what we consume could be the answer to so many problems. But while these connections could be the answer for our own health and wellbeing, we also need to recognise the connections that exist between the problems in the wider world.

What would be the point in being vegan for the animals, if we aren't considering the exploitation, displacement and killing of fellow humans because of the food industry? Or being vegan to save animals *and* humans, whilst our home is burning. And why would we eat a seemingly ethical vegan diet which goes on to harm our health, so that we can no longer advocate effectively for the oppressed?

Of course you could find other diets that are almost as healthy, like the Mediterranean diet, but they just aren't as good for the planet when they still include meat and dairy, and they certainly are not as good for animal equality and rights. For example, somebody who is recommending a plant-based diet for health could probably argue that a small amount of fish would be a healthful choice, and they wouldn't be entirely wrong. But when we consider the impact that this has on the climate, the oceans, and on the fish themselves, it no longer remains a serious suggestion.

With our growing population and dying planet, there really is only one choice for the future of humanity, and that's to learn how to live kinder and more compassionately. The only choice is veganism.

I hope you can see, however, that despite what we've all been led to believe about how we shop, cook, eat and live, it really is easier to live a plant-rich life than you previously imagined. It really isn't about what you will leave behind, but instead is about opening your mind and heart to a whole different way of living. Get started, and I promise you will never look back.

Useful Resources

Books

Eating Plant-Based: Scientific answers to your nutrition questions. Dr Shireen Kassam and Dr Zahra Kassam, 17th February 2022, Hammersmith Health Books. ISBN-10 1781611947

How to Argue with a Meat Eater (and Win Every Time). Ed Winters, 19th December 2024, Vermilion. ISBN-10 1785044494

How not to Age: The Scientific Approach to Getting Healthier as You Get Older. Michael Greger, 7th December 2023, Bluebird. ISBN-10 1529057353

How Not to Die. Michael Greger and Gene Stone, 28th December 2017, Pan. ISBN-10 1509852506

Plant-Based Nutrition in Clinical Practice. Dr Shireen Kassam, Dr Zahra Kassam and Lisa Simon RD, 15th September 2022, Hammersmith Health Books. 178161198X

Finding Me in Menopause: Flourishing in Perimenopause and Menopause using Nutrition and Lifestyle. Dr Nitu Bajekal, Rohini Bajekal and Rajiv Bajeka, 25/04/2024, Sheldon Press. ISBN-10 1399810227

The Plant-Based Diet Revolution: 28 Days to a Happier Gut and a Healthier You. Dr Alan Desmond and Bob Andrew, 7th January 2021, Yellow Kite. ISBN-10 1529308682

The Plant Power Doctor: A Simple Prescription for a Healthier You. Dr Gemma Newman, 7th January 2021, Ebury Press. ISBN-10 1529107741

The Science of Plant-Based Nutrition: How to Enhance the Power of Plants for Optimal Health. Rhiannon Lambert, 27th June 2024, DK. ISBN-10 024166876X

This Is Vegan Propaganda (And other lies the meat industry tells you). Ed Winters, 5th January 2023, Vermilion. ISBN-10 1785044249

Ultra-Processed People. Dr Chris Van Tulleken, 2nd May 2024, Penguin. ISBN-10 1529160227

Films

I have to admit that I haven't watched all of these, but I know these are the films that come highly recommended by vegans for helping you to commit to the cause. I find the health/planet related films really useful for bolstering my own knowledge, or finding ways to explain the arguments for veganism to other people. As for the animal rights based movies, they're the ones I just can't bring myself to watch. If you want to be persuaded that we shouldn't be farming, slaughtering and eating animals, particularly on the scale that we are doing so, then I suggest you give them a go. But as I'm already thoroughly convinced that the animal agriculture industry is wrong, I have chosen not to put myself through the trauma of seeing it all unfold on a screen in front of me.

Cowspiracy, 2014

Dominion, 2018

Earthlings, 2015

I Could Never Go Vegan, 2024

Seaspiracy, 2021

What the Health, 2017

Websites

The Vegan Doctor – www.thevegandoctor.co.uk

The Vegan Society – www.vegansociety.com

Plant-Based Health Professionals UK_– www.plantbasedhealthprofessionals.com

Physicians Committee for Responsible Medicine – www.pcrm.org

Nutrition Facts – www.nutritionfact.org

Viva! The Vegan Charity – www.viva.org.uk

Glossary

Adipocytes – fat cells

Adipokines – cell signalling proteins released by adipocytes

Amines – a nitrogen-containing organic compound

Anaemia – haemoglobin level of <130g/L in men, and <120g/L in non-pregnant women

Androgens – hormone that regulates the development and maintenance of typically male sexual characteristics

Angina – exertional chest pain that results from partially occluded coronary arteries

Anticapitalism – a political ideology and movement that opposes capitalism

Antioxidants – naturally occurring chemicals that prevent oxidation, a biological process that results in harmful free radicals

Atheroma – a fatty plaque that can block blood vessels

Atherosclerosis – the process of narrowing and hardening of blood vessels which are occluded by atheromas

Bile acids – molecules that are made in the liver, and help to digest fats and regular cholesterol

Bioavailability – how well a substance can be absorbed

Biodiversity – the variety and variability of life on earth

Biofuels – fuels made from plants, animals, or waste

Breast(/chest)feeding – used to describe both breastfeeding and chestfeeding, where the latter describes how transgender and non-binary parents describe feeding an infant their own milk from their chest

Butyrate – a short-chain fatty acid produced by gut bacteria, which has health benefits

Calorie density – the number of calories in a given volume of food

Cardiovascular disease – disease that affects the heart and blood vessels, usually referring to the blockage of these with atheromatous plaques

Carotid arteries – blood vessels that supply the brain with oxygenated blood

Cervix – the neck of the womb

Cholesterol – a waxy substance, used in the body to make hormones and bile, amongst other processes

Chronic kidney disease – disease of the kidney which causes reduced function

Class 1 carcinogen – a substance known to cause cancer in humans

Class 2 carcinogen – a substance thought to probably cause cancer in humans

Cognitive dissonance – the mental disturbance felt when a person's beliefs and actions don't align

Cohort study – a type of observational study that follows a group of participants over a period of time

Crohn's disease – one of the types of inflammatory bowel disease

DASH diet – the Dietary Approaches to Stop Hypertension diet was developed to help manage hypertension

Deforestation – removal and destruction of forest land to convert it to non-forest use

Delerium – acute confusion, often seen in the elderly, due to a medical cause

Deoxycholic acid – one of the secondary bile acids

Dexa scan – a low dose x-ray that measures bone density

Diverticular disease – the formation of abnormal pouches in the colon

Diverticula – the pouches that occur in the bowel in diverticular disease

Diverticulitis – inflammation of the diverticula

Euthanised – deliberately having ended a life for the purpose of ending suffering

Factory farming – an intensive method of farming to maximise production for the least cost

Ferritin – a protein inside the body's cells that stores iron

Fibre – a type of carbohydrate that isn't digested in the small intestine, so reaches the colon intact

Fortified – having healthy substances added

Free-range eggs – eggs from hens that are not kept in cages

Gaseous exchange – the process of oxygen passing from the lungs into the bloodstream, and CO_2 waste passing the opposite way to be breathed out

Ghost gear – lost and abandoned fishing equipment

Global warming – the increase in global average temperature, probably due to human activities

Glomerulus – a collection of blood vessels in the kidney which filters blood plasma

Glomerular filtration rate – the measure of filtration in the kidney, which describes how well the kidney is working

Glycaemic index (GI) – a score given to a food to describe how quickly and to what extent is causes the blood sugar to rise after eating it

Greenhouse gases – gases in the atmosphere that increase the earth's surface temperature

Growth factors – proteins or hormones that stimulate cell proliferation and wound healing (IGF-1 is insulin-like growth factor-1, a growth factor and type of hormone, similar to insulin, which is important in growth in children, and in high levels is associated with some cancers)

Haem – the iron containing part of haemoglobin, which binds oxygen in the bloodstream

Haemoglobin – a protein that contains iron, and transports oxygen in red blood cells

HDL – high density lipoprotein

Heterocyclic amines – chemical compounds, some of which are carcinogenic and produced when meat is cooked at a high temperature

Hidradenitis suppurativa – a skin condition which involves boils, abscesses and sinuses

Hormone replacement therapy (HRT) – medication used to treat hormone deficiencies, for example in the menopause

Hyperandrogenism – the state of high blood androgen levels

Hypercholesterolaemia – blood levels of cholesterol that are higher than the normal reference range

Hyperkalaemia – high blood potassium levels

Hypokalaemia – low blood potassium levels

Hyponatraemia – low blood sodium levels

Indigenous – naturally existing in a place, rather than arriving from another place

Industrialisation – a period of social and economic change from farming to the use of technology to mass produce

Insemination – the introduction of sperm into a female reproductive system to fertilise an ovum

Insulin – a hormone, produced by the pancreas, which promotes the absorption of glucose from the bloodstream into cells

Insulin resistance – a state in which cells don't respond well to insulin, so don't absorb glucose from the blood

Insulin sensitivity – how well the body's cells respond to insulin

Ischaemic heart disease – a condition in which the heart is affected by blocked arteries, resulting in angina and myocardial infarction

Isoflavones – a type of phytoestrogen, found in high quantities in soya beans

Keto – referring to the 'ketogenic diet', one which prioritises fats, reduces protein, and minimises carbohydrate intake. Used by some people for weight loss, but it has other medical uses

Lactase – an enzyme produced in the guts of mammals to break down the sugar, lactose, found in milk

Lactose – a sugar found in milk

Lanolin – a wax found in the wool of animals, such as sheep

LDL-C – low-density lipoprotein cholesterol is cholesterol that is carried by low density lipoproteins, which is associated with an increased risk of cardiovascular disease

LGBTQ+ – lesbian, gay, bisexual, transsexual and queer, encompassing all sexualities and gender identities that are not cis heterosexual

Macrocytosis – a description of the situation in which red blood cells are enlarged, usually caused by deficiency or disease

MASLD – metabolic dysfunction-associated steatotic liver disease, describing excessive fat storage in the liver associated with other metabolic problems such as insulin resistance and obesity

Mastitis – inflammation of the breast or udder, usually associated with breast(/chest)feeding

Mediterranean diet – a diet inspired by the cuisine of Greece and southern Italy, centred around plant-based eating, unprocessed grains, fruits, vegetables, fruits and legumes. It does include oily fish, small amounts of meat, and moderate intake of alcohol

Menopause – the time when periods stop and fertility ceases

Meta-analysis – a method of data production, combining results from lots of studies

Metabolic syndrome – the state of having at least three of the following: abdominal obesity; raised blood pressure; raised fasting blood sugar; raised blood triglyceride levels; and low blood levels of HDL-C

Microbiome – community of microbes living in any given habitat, but usually referring to those within the human body, for example the gut microbiome

Microcytosis – smaller than usual red cells, also often caused by deficiency, usually of iron.

Micronutrients – essential dietary elements, required by the human body for various biological processes

Microplastics – pieces of plastic <5mm long

Myocardial infarction – the medical name for a heart attack

Neurodevelopmental disorders – mental conditions affecting development of the nervous system

Neurotransmitters – the chemicals which are released by one nerve and received by another, creating a signal

Nitrates and nitrites – food additives put into meat to enhance flavour and improve longevity, which can be converted to carcinogenic compounds

N-nitroso compounds – harmful substances produced by presence of nitrates and nitrites in foods

Obesity – a body mass index (BMI) of >30kg/m

Omnivorous – describing somebody who follows a diet that doesn't restrict animal products

Osteoblasts/osteoclasts – the cells in bone tissue that build, break down and remodel bones

Osteopenia – the state of under-mineralised bone, causing thinning, or reduced bone mass

Osteoporosis – a step on from osteopenia, this is more severe thinning of the bones, associated with fractures

Phenols/polyphenols – chemical compounds produced by plants and microorganisms, and have antioxidant properties

Phytosterols/sterols/stanols – phtyosterols are compounds from plants, and include sterols and stanols. They have positive effects on LDL levels

PITS – perpetration induced traumatic stress, occurring when PTSD symptoms occur after being involved in a violent act

Pituitary gland – a small gland that sits just beneath the brain and releases several different hormones

Plant-based – eating a diet of mostly plants

Postprandial – describing the bodily state after eating

Primary prevention – preventing a disease before it occurs

PTSD – post-traumatic stress disorder, a mental disorder arising from a traumatic event

Premature death – death between ages 30 and 70 years, usually referring to those from cardiovascular diseases, cancer, diabetes, and chronic respiratory diseases

Processed meat – meat that has been modified to improve its flavour or shelf-life

PUFA – polyunsaturated fatty acids, the precursors to polyunsaturated fats

Rheumatoid arthritis – an inflammatory type of arthritis, due to autoimmune disease

Ruminants – grazing animals which ferment their food in the stomach in order to extract nutrition

Saturated fat – a sub-type of fat which is usually found in animal proteins and is associated with an increased risk of cardiovascular disease

Secondary prevention – reducing the impact of a disease once it has occurred

Stoma – an opening created in the abdominal wall to allow the excretion of stools when surgery means that the rectum can no longer be used

Thermic effect – the amount of energy used, above the basal metabolic rate, for the processing of food during digestion

Thyroid gland – a gland sitting in the front of the neck, which produces thyroid hormone, which controls our metabolic rate

TMAO – Trimethylamine N-oxide, a metabolite from red meat digestion, which is associated with cardiovascular disease

Trans fats – a type of unsaturated fat, which is usually artificially synthesised, and has harmful effects on the body. They have been banned in some countries

Triglycerides – the main constituents of body fats in humans, and in excess can have harmful effects on human health

Ulcerative colitis – one of the types of inflammatory bowel disease

Ultraprocessed foods – a category of food classified within the NOVA classification system to describe industrially manufactured foods which contain food substance of no or rare culinary use

Unsaturated fat – another sub-type of fat, and along with poly- and monounsaturated and unsaturated fats, are known as the good fats, because they are not associated with an increased risk in cardiovascular disease, and have some health benefits

Veal – flesh from a calf aged from a few hours old up to around 35 weeks old

Vegan – someone who follows a lifestyle that avoids products which have been derived from or involved the exploitation of non-human (and human) animals

Vegetarian – somebody who follows a diet which doesn't contain meat or fish, but they do consume eggs and dairy

Weaning – the period of taking a young child or animal off their mother's milk and onto solid foods instead

WFPB – whole-food plant-based, describing a plant-based diet where foods are only consumed when 'whole' and minimally processed

References

**Scan the QR code for access to
references**

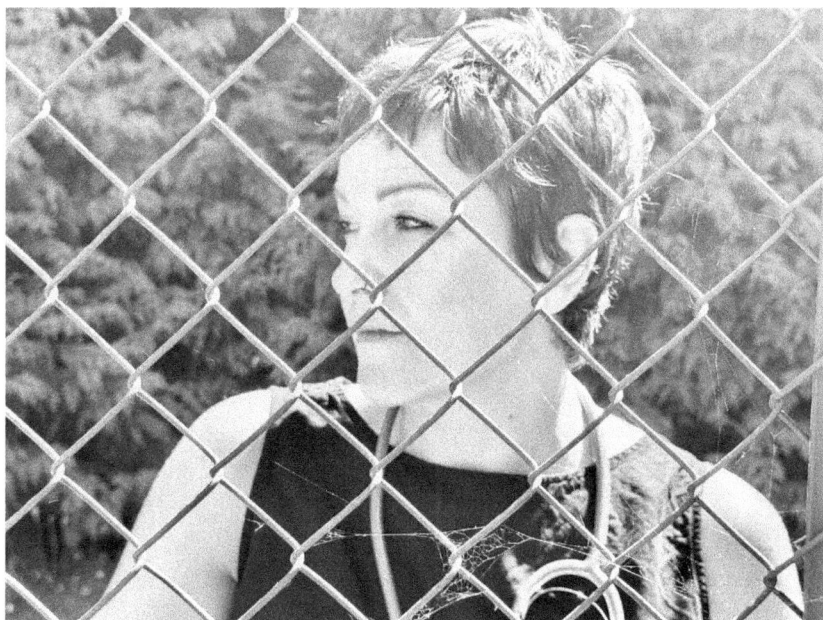

Image by Maria Slough Photography

Dr Rebecca E. Jones is a GP, writer, activist and mum, living and working in London. She has been writing The Vegan Doctor blog since 2017, and her articles have been featured in The Guardian, The Telegraph, i, and many other publications. As well as her medical training, Rebecca has a postgraduate diploma in Clinical Nutrition, and is working towards her Lifestyle Medicine diploma. Whilst becoming vegan was initially an ethical choice for the rights of animals, her reading and research has led her to believe that plant-based eating is also essential to safeguard the future health of humanity, and to protect the earth and all of its inhabitants. Rebecca incorporates plant-based nutrition advice in her day-to-day encounters with NHS patients, and enjoys educating colleagues about the benefits of plant-dominant diets. She is the founder of the Facebook group Vegan Doctors of the UK, and a member of Plant Based Health Professionals UK. Rebecca keeps an entirely vegan household for her two young children.